IT HAPPENED TO ME

Gidske Anderson is a successful Norwegian journalist and author whose writing career began in the underground press during the German occupation of Norway in World War II. She has been Vice-President of the Norwegian Nobel Committee, which annually awards the Nobel Peace Prize, since 1982.

Gidske Anderson

IT HAPPENED
TO ME

Translated by Joan Tate

Futura

A Futura Book

Copyright © Gyldendal Norsk Forlag A/S 1983

Copyright © this translation Joan Tate 1986

Originally published by Gyldendal Norsk Forlag,
Oslo, 1983, under the title: *Det hendte meg*

First published in Great Britain in 1986
by Futura Publications, a Division of
Macdonald & Co (Publishers) Ltd
London & Sydney

ISBN 0 7088 2975 9

Typeset in Times by Fleet Graphics, Enfield, Middlesex

Printed in Great Britain by The Guernsey Press

Futura Publications
A Division of
Macdonald & Company (Publishers) Ltd
Greater London House
Hampstead Road
London NW1 7QX

A BPCC plc Company

Chapter One

It had never occurred to me that it could happen to me. On the whole, I have never even given such matters a thought, possibly because I have always been too occupied with other things. I see myself now, in retrospect, charging ahead at top speed through the landscape. There's a river to wade across, and I wade away across it. Then – in the middle of the turbulent waters, standing knee-deep – it happens.

What is it that happens? One day I am standing in my bath, literally standing in the bath and looking at myself in the mirror. I see that my right breast has something unfamiliar about it, something puckered about the nipple. At that very moment, I see in front of me a photograph in some newspaper urging women to keep a watch on their breasts. The condition shown on the photograph was one that needed consultation with a doctor.

I must admit I pushed that possibility out of my

mind at first. I'll think about it tomorrow . . . Some time went by like that – a relatively short time, I would say. But every morning as I was taking a bath I looked at myself, until one day it was *imperative* that another person should look at that breast, and then the reaction was spontaneous. Go and see your doctor!

I went to the doctor the next day. He had been my doctor for a long time, and I had had sporadic contact with him for many years. 'You have a growth,' he said, and 'The growth will have to be examined by specialists.'

'You mean I've got cancer?'

'I didn't say that. I can't answer that question.'

'Are there growths that aren't cancer, then?'

'There are lots of different kinds of harmless growths, yes.'

My own doctor *couldn't* tell me if it was cancer. I know that. Formally and in reality, he was not able to. But I didn't believe him at the time. I thought there was something in his look. But most of all, I now had my own forebodings. For the first time, in all its reality, I realized it was likely I had cancer in my right breast.

That was one day at the end of February in 1983. When I left my doctor's surgery, I looked at the world with different eyes. I walked slowly along the streets. I walked along Geitemyr Road past St Hans Langen and took the Ulleval Road into the city.

The tall trees along St Hansheugen; I fixed my eyes on them and followed their proud trunks, their black branches splayed out against a low grey February sky. Everything was grey or black. The picture stuck, grew,

8

and filled me. Slowly the picture of the black trunks and branches against a grey sky arose in my mind and imprinted itself there. It will be there always.

I walked on slowly into the city. I was in no hurry. Neither was there any haste within me. As if from a distance from myself, I registered the way in which I slowed down the pace I had probably kept up for many years. A pace that had been quite natural, in as much as I had liked it, because I liked my work. And at that particular period, I was absorbed in work on a book that took up nearly all my time.

I could hear my own steps going more and more slowly along the road and I could feel the blood in my veins also slowing down. A great cold emptiness slowly descended on me. A feeling of having abandoned something. As if, as I left my doctor's surgery, I had sailed away in a large black boat, on a long solo journey. As if I had put most things behind me.

I crossed Ulleval Road. I went into an antiquarian bookshop and lost myself for half an hour among the shelves there. But first of all, I took the opportunity to pay a bill I had not settled.

I had an appointment that day with Tim Greve, the editor of the newspaper *Verdens Gang* (The Way of the World). I was going to ask him for some information in connection with the book I was working on, and I was also going to tell him whether I would be able to give a lecture in the early summer, as he had suggested. I'll 'phone him from a kiosk, I thought, and tell him I've been delayed. A little further on into the city, I changed my mind. I would meet him at the agreed time. There was no reason to stop living. Better to float along on the current of the day, as long as there was something to float on.

I had an hour before I was to meet Greve. I walked slowly on. I passed Norli's bookshop in University Street and remembered I had once noticed a medical department at the back of the shop. I went in. I looked aimlessly along categories and titles and finally came to the section of books on nursing. There I found a hardback book of about two hundred pages, with a large dark-blue crab on the jacket. The book was Danish and entitled *The Treatment and Care of Cancer Patients*.

I suppose I am what they call a bookworm. But books on diseases, medical books and health books have not played a large part in my life, and those I have read had nothing to do with me. I haven't been ill for thirty-seven years, and that was an infectious disease I caught when travelling in post-war Europe.

Now I was standing there with a book on cancer in my hand. And the book concerned *me*. A quick leaf through it showed me it had a chapter on breast cancer. I bought it, put it in my bag and went off to my meeting with Tim Greve. We went out to lunch together at The Bristol.

It was an unusually pleasant meal. Tim Greve comes from Bergen. I have known him for at least thirty years and both our brief as well as our slightly longer meetings over all those years have always taken on the nature of a party. People from Bergen bring with them happiness, humour and enthusiasm. They are probably no happier than the rest of us. But I suppose they are the only urbane creatures among our slow, inarticulate and melancholy countrymen. I like the style of Bergen people immensely, perhaps because they remind me a little of Parisians, whom I have lived among for so many years.

10

We had stories to tell each other, Greve and I, amusing, even uproarious stories. I said a few words to him as we were putting our coats on before leaving: I would tell him in a week's time whether I could give that lecture he had suggested. I said I had an 'examination on the go' and would telephone him as soon as things were settled.

We parted with a smile. I heard him behind me as I stood on the pavement and was just about to cross the street: 'Take care of yourself, Gidske,' with a Bergen breeziness in his voice. I turned round and nodded to him, smiling too. Good old Tim, if only it was in my power to do so.

But at the moment there was little I could do. I had basically just been told to wait. I had been 'referred' by my doctor to Ullevål hospital for further examination and I would hear from them. It was three days before I received a written note giving me an appointment five days later.

A week in a vacuum. I swung between wild optimism, a relatively normal reaction in me, and profound pessimism, a rather new and disquieting feeling. One moment I thought: it is only what they call in the cancer book a 'benign' growth in the breast. They would remove it and that would be that. But the next moment, the barbaric descriptions would strike me like thunderbolts: the 'primary tumour' in the breast could turn out to be 'malign', in other words breast-cancer. In addition to that, 'lymph nodule metastases' could be involved, and also 'secondary metastases' that could spread to different internal organs.

Again and again, I read those chilling explanations. A vacant but persistent uncertainty descended on my days and nights. I knew only one thing for certain, and that was what my doctor had explained to me. No one could say anything definite until they had taken out a section of the growth in my breast and had it analysed.

I was in no state to do any sensible work. But my tax declaration for 1982 was due to be handed in before the first of March. I buried myself in columns of figures, studying the regulations and doing lengthy calculations. All those figures and paragraphs kept other thoughts at a distance. It was my first exercise in pure will-power, trying to chase the whole cancer business out of my head. I managed to, time and time again, thanks to Norway's incredibly complicated tax system.

On Wednesday, the second of March, at two o'clock, I went to the Surgical Unit at Ullevål hospital to take up my appointment, as the note instructed. I took a taxi. It was raining as I drove in through the entrance to Ullevål.

I don't think I have seen that entrance since 1946, when at the age of twenty-five, I was in Ullevål for a complicated tooth operation. I looked round now with a sleep-walker's guardedness at the old area. There were large trees there, too, with which I have always connected Ullevål ever since I was a child. Tall black trunks, bare black branches, again those elegant etchings against a low grey sky. Everywhere people in white clothes coming and going, and what I remembered as a large park now had cars parked all over it. Great modern buildings had appeared in several places, and I knew nothing about them. The old Ullevål buildings were touching remnants of the past in this world of concrete, glass and cars.

THANK YOU FOR
SHOPPING AT

THE NEW *Lewis's*

THANK YOU FOR
SHOPPING AT

```
312601    1 0214 01031    21APR6

PAPERBACKS
386                     1      1.95

                      TOTAL    1.95


BUY WITH A LEWISS MONTHLY A C
```

The cab-driver knew where to go and took me to the correct entrance. A glass door. A corridor, full of busy women and men. Into another, inner corridor, over to a hatchway into an office. Then sitting waiting in a long light passage together with a great many others.

My turn came at last. A fair-haired, friendly sister received me and asked me to strip to the waist. The doctor would be coming, she said in a gentle, quiet voice, then disappeared. I looked round: it was a large, light and modern room, rather bare and empty but there was a high examination couch in the middle of the floor.

I undressed and sat down on a chair. The consultant came, a calm, subdued man, followed by a shy younger man, who turned out to be a medical student. The doctor examined my breast and the growth.

I had entered a different and self-absorbing world. From then on, a magic circle was thrown round me, invisible but powerfully strong.

Light and spotlessly clean corridors, steady streams of white-clad people, brief glimpses of huge apparatus. This quiet subdued world, and the contrast between the two worlds – on the one side white-clad young men and women, healthy, handsome, clean and gentle, and on the other the sick, the *bent* and shaken, the burnt-out or shattered, sometimes pushed along a corridor on a wheeled bed, but also sitting in long rows in the waiting-corridor, each sunk in his or her own illness.

Or sitting alone in a consulting room, just as I was.

The doctor felt the lump with experienced fingers and said something in a low voice to the medical student, who was observing quietly and intently, smiling politely at me. After a while, the doctor sat back in his chair and gave me a calm and comprehensive explanation.

He did not have to explain that I had a growth, but there was the suspicion that it might be malignant. However, that could only be verified by surgical intervention, in which an incision was made in the breast, the growth removed and then analysed. This analysis would take place while I was under the anaesthetic. Should the tumour be malignant, the surgeon would have to take the decision there and then whether to remove my right breast. They would have no opportunity to consult me. So I had to agree to this beforehand.

It was as simple as that, all said in quiet tones, with a kindness that was probably professional, but also betrayed a natural humanity. When I think back on this scene, I still break out in a cold sweat and a wave of something I would quite simply call grief surges up inside me. But at the time, I was empty, cold, beyond this world.

'I would like to do a more thorough examination . . .' The doctor said something of the kind as he rose and asked me to get on to the examination couch. Professional hands 'palpated' (as it says in the nursing book on cancer) various parts of me. A section was also taken from the growth in my breast.

The doctor was standing over me, his back concealing my breast. I said nothing. But I felt it. They cut into me. Cutting out the section really hurt what I still thought of as my healthy body. A large plaster was

14

put over the incision, a brilliant white flower on the upper part of my breast. I got up and put on my clothes, then sat down on the very edge of a chair, straight as a poker.

The doctor spoke to the sister, saying it would be best done as soon as possible. 'Don't you think so?' he said, turning to me. I nodded. Sister suggested the beginning of the following week. The doctor interrupted and said, 'We'll do it on Friday,' turning enquiringly to me. I nodded.

'Can you arrange that, Sister?' I heard him say, and she arranged it. I left the room with several bits of paper in my hand. One for a blood-test. Another for an X-ray, and an A4 size paper on which the following was printed with the relevant information in handwriting:

You have been allocated a bed in the Surgical Unit, Ward 23 on Friday, 4th March, 1983. You are requested to follow the instructions below:

You are asked to present yourself at Surgical Reception at 7.00 hours having fasted, i.e. having not eaten, drunk, smoked or chewed chewing-gum after 24.00 hours the previous day.

The chewing-gum made me laugh. I don't think I have chewed gum since I used to play hopscotch in Oslo fifty years ago. But what harm could chewing-gum do before an operation?

I knew nothing. I knew absolutely nothing about what an anaesthetic entailed. The only operation I had ever had was when I had my appendix out when I was nine years old. My memory of the anaesthetic then was a feeling of being suffocated. I had no idea whatsoever what was going to happen now, apart from the fact that everyone assured me that 'anaesthetics were quite different these days'. And 'everyone' – they were friends and acquaintances. The amazing thing was that I didn't ask anyone at the hospital. But I was empty, a dutiful person being obedient, mutely following the instructions I had been given.

That first day inside the magic circle, like a sheep, unquestioning I took my papers to the various departments. To blood-tests; resigned, I ascertained that my veins were 'deep' or awkwardly placed, just as they always had been. I loathe injections or needles being jabbed into me. Sister stuck the needle in only a few times before she found the vein. I stared absentmindedly at the blood she divided up into various small tubes.

On to the X-ray. As I stood stripped to the waist in front of the huge X-ray apparatus, the sister said: 'You've been here before, haven't you?' I smiled bleakly and just said no. I realized she had recognized my face from a newspaper photograph or from television, but I hadn't the energy to explain to her. But she persisted. She looked at my papers and smiled broadly: 'You're the one in Paris, aren't you?' 'Have been,' I said tamely.

The sister was gentle, friendly, full of interest, one of the many good people I was to meet inside that magic circle in the months ahead. I tried to smile back as best I could, but I was fundamentally abstracted from everyone. I was *no one*. I was empty. A sheep in a flock of sheep. I observed myself, as if standing to one side of myself. I was surprised. There seemed to be

16

no connection at all between the sheep I was and *me*.

Almost as if in a panic, the faintest suspicion arose. I fought to keep some kind of control over something that was rising within me, more and more evidently as the routine examinations went on. This was clearly anguish.

An all-embracing darkness lay ahead of me and dutifully, I continued in that direction. 'Like a lamb to slaughter!' I thought, almost saying it aloud here and there in those long passages full of white-clad, fit and beautiful nurses.

I got a hold on myself as I left the hospital that day. I had been granted about forty hours before I was due back again in the Surgical Unit. I kept myself in an iron grip that day, and escaped under that glass bell of iron will.

Escaping from the anguish. The tumour would surely turn out to be benign when they operated. All the small practical things that had to be arranged – appointments cancelled, work postponed, friends and acquaintances told. That was also an escape. On the first evening of my forty hour portion of time, I had a good meal in good company and drank a bottle of first class French red wine. And I drank myself silly after the meal.

But all through my panicky attempts to escape, the anguish grew unabated. By the end of the time, I had admitted to myself the fact that my breast would be removed. I really was going to the slaughter.

I have worked to deadlines all my adult life. So I am a precise person, always arriving slightly early for fear of being late. I took the same precautions on Friday the fourth of March. Not trusting the alarm clock, I booked a telephone alarm call and ordered a

17

taxi for quarter past six, to be on the safe side, so there would be no danger of arriving too late.

My old ME observed this new ME. Extraordinary creature, I said. Here you are on your way down towards what suspiciously resembled what the Greeks called dark Hades, and you are making elaborate preparations as if for a holiday.

That was the only way I could keep myself under some kind of control – the security of definite times, of an organized schedule that would give me enough time to have a leisurely bath and a calm departure from my apartment. The mechanism worked. I went to bed relatively early on that last evening and slept like a child, a whole night's sleep without even an aspirin to send me off.

The next morning was dark and rainy. I could hear the sound of my own steps on the stairs, and by the time I was only one flight down I could hear the taxi outside waiting for me, its engine running.

The ride to Ullevål Hospital did not take long in the empty morning streets. I was sitting up straight in the back, my eyes following the contours of the city we were driving through. As I have thought so many times in my life, I thought about how much I liked Queen's Park. I made a mental note, that in the great avenue of lime trees, which many generations ago had once led to a small pavilion, the tall trees that March morning were not showing the slightest sign of spring.

We drove past the slopes down to the duck pond in the Palace Park. I thought about my very first ski-run down a hill. Park Road, behind me. Past the first building in that street, also part of my childhood, where my grandmother lived somewhere on the upper storeys. And then Bislet Sports Stadium, to me always a picture of gloom. Then up Therese Street, endless Therese Street, grey and anonymous. Then in through the entrance of the hospital.

Those big old trees again, bare and black on a grey wet morning. Down the ramp to the Surgical Unit. Pay the taxi-driver. Out with my suitcase, containing the regulation 'Toilet articles, dressing-gown, slippers and socks' as my admission papers said, and don't forget the 'urine sample' (morning).

The taxi drove away, and there I was with my suitcase. It was only about half past six. I was half an hour too early. I just stood there looking round rather irresolutely at this thoroughly impersonal place, a tunnel through which cars drove straight in and straight out again after delivering patients. I saw someone inside a rather shabby communal glass door. I had to go in. I did.

I was met by a handsome man who said good-morning to me. I held out my admission papers and said apologetically that I was not supposed to come until seven o'clock. That was perfectly all right. I could just sit down and wait. I sat down in a room and waited. The man came in with a morning paper and said, 'Perhaps you'd like to take a look at the paper while you're waiting?' And I looked at the paper. Then another person came in, a young girl with a suitcase in her hand, just like me. She came in quietly, as I had done. We said good-morning to each other. Then we sat there waiting.

A sister came in shortly after seven. She had a batch of

19

papers in her hand and asked for 'Anderson'. She took me into a small bare room where there was a bed on wheels, made up, splendid and white.

When I saw it, I thought: 'How on earth will I manage to get into that bed?' But the sister knew her job. I was to hang my coat and hat there, she said, and had I been through my coat pockets? Then she whirled me through a mass of papers, information and registrations.

My sheep-like nature came stealing back over me. As dutifully as a 1930s girl, just like in the days when schoolchildren held up their hands in class and never said a word before the teacher had nodded in confirmation, I dutifully filled up a form, signed it and answered the questions.

Then I had to undress. Sister handed me a large pair of wide knee-pants made of sweet-smelling linen, together with an equally large smock. I got them on eventually. Just before I crawled into that bed in the middle of the room, I caught a glimpse of a man quietly coming in and putting labels on my coat and hat.

Then there was much bustling round me. Nurses came and went, speaking quietly to each other, and 'my' sister said something about she was going to give me an injection now because they were in a hurry – 'you have to be ready by eight o'clock.'

Good, I thought, now you're off. I was lying as stiff as a board under the quilt, feeling like the trunk of a felled tree more than anything else. But the injection was working. A feeling of calm indifference was stealing over me. Then a nurse came in and said something like, 'Well, off we go, then!' And off we went out through the door.

Through other doors that opened automatically. Down long passages, and round a corner. The bed stopped there. 'My' doctor came over to me, the one who had examined me two days earlier. He was wearing what must have been 'operating clothes' and had a small skullcap on his head. He said: 'Good-morning, Gidske Anderson. I will be carrying out your operation.' He reminded me of the explanation he had given me two days ago, clarifying the course of action and asking me whether I had understood what was going to happen.

I nodded. I don't think I said a word. What could I say? The injection was working so that I was regarding all life and surroundings with a benevolent indifference.

That is the last thing I remember clearly.

From then on, fog enveloped everything and I slowly vanished into total darkness. I remember nothing but the bed moving on and I had a faint sense of going up in a large lift, then into a large open room where there were a great many busy white-clad people. And I distinctly remember very clearly an older, very nice sister who . . . well, who what? That has vanished into the black darkness that now came down like a curtain.

It is an amazing experience losing ten or twelve hours out of your life. When I was twenty-five, I had a feverish illness, during which I was what they call unconscious for several days. I had very intense, feverish dreams, quite unconnected with reality but very relevant in my mind. I remember those days vividly; they were more real than many actual events in my life. I still remember them today, thirty-five years later.

But those ten or twelve hours of the fourth of March, 1983, have gone. NOTHING. I lived for half that day in NOTHING. All attempts to recapture them have been in vain. I tried to get a doctor to explain to me, purely physiologically, what actually happens in such situations, but he remarked rather dryly that it was no more remarkable than when one slept at night.

I have thought it over, and it is true. I can recapture very little indeed of my sleep the morning after, even if it is possible at times. But I also have a feeling that by concentrating hard, I should gradually be able to get into myself within the realm of sleep.

But that fourth of March, 1983, is as if sliced out of my life. Black. Cold. Like an iron wall.

It must have been about six in the evening that day when I came drifting out of a dark world of fog, hovering weightlessly, a transparent, gauzy creature, sailing out of the darkness.

Then I registered that I was lying in bed. I was naked, surrounded by white curtains and with great white pillows under my head. Above my bed was some apparatus from which a kind of tube ran down to my left wrist and also to another part of my body. The outline of a man's head appeared out of the dark on my right.

I heard a voice say: 'Can you hear me now?' I could, so I nodded. Quietly, the voice told me they had had to remove my right breast.

I could feel the whole of my right side held in the

firm grasp of large bandages. I was thirsty and asked for water, but there was no response to my request. White shadows flitted round me, and after a while I managed to focus sufficiently to see it was a nurse, or several nurses.

I again asked for some water. My mouth was as dry as dust and I felt as if I were choking. The nurse came with a stick with cotton-wool on it and stuck it into my mouth. It was soaked in mint or something like that and set my saliva glands into action, so the worst of my thirst disappeared very soon. I heard the sister ask if I were feeling sick. I thought about it – no, I was not feeling sick. I was just thirsty, as I kept saying.

I must have fallen asleep, or I vanished back into the darkness again, then came back to the bed and the semi-dark room under the impression that someone was moving round me.

The person closest to me in my life was sitting on the edge of my bed. I looked up and could find only one thing to say: 'They've cut off my right breast.'

A nurse came in with a large bouquet of roses and put it on my locker. She handed me an envelope. I took it with both hands and registered surprise that I was able to use my right hand as well. I was rather stiff down my right side but had no real pain. I managed to open the envelope quite easily, and read the card: 'Gidske dear. Love from us all. Andreas.'

It was from my publisher.

Then I returned to the darkness again, or rather I floated weightlessly back into a sort of semi-dark world.

I was woken by someone pushing my bed, out of

the door, down along an endless corridor, into another department. My bed was put against a wall in a passage and I heard two nurses discussing where a space could be found for me. They could not agree on the subject because I was left lying there along the wall. But then a young energetic nurse came along and I heard her say: 'I've got a place.' The bed was pushed further down the passage and into a ward.

I was thirsty. I was overwhelmingly thirsty. Basically, nothing else existed for me, just this thirst, thirst, thirst. A sister came and put a screen round my bed. Again, I asked for something to drink.

She brought the same little stick, and that helped a little, for a while. She also asked if I were feeling sick. But no, I was only thirsty. Then she quietly told me that I would probably not be allowed anything to drink until early the next morning. That sounded so impossible, I went on saying I was thirsty.

Yes, I was pitiable. My thirst did indeed over-shadow everything, but otherwise I felt endlessly wretched in every way – vulnerable, not really fright-ened, but helpless. Like a speck of dust.

Then the nurse was back again, arranging the curtains, helping me into a position in bed that allowed my body to rest and fixing pillows so that my stiff arm and the stiff side of my torso were comfortable.

I couldn't see her face, which melted into the semi-darkness, but I heard her low voice. I have seldom felt such helpless gratitude surging through me towards a totally unknown person.

I heard her ask me if I was comfortable, and I actually was, so I nodded. She probably again told me I couldn't have any water until tomorrow morning and she gave me another mint-stick, saying very quietly that I was going to be given something to make me sleep. And I was.

Slowly, I sank into sleep, in a surprisingly secure and almost comforted mood.

The next morning, I woke up in a ward where there turned out to be five other patients. I was eventually given something to drink and eat, and that gave me a positive feeling of well-being. I had no pain – at least none to speak of. The whole of my right side was indeed stiff, and I had some difficulty moving both my arm and shoulder, but the generous arrangement of pillows that sister helped me with made up for a great deal.

I had woken very early that morning, and in the semi-darkness I watched the gradually increasing activity of the nurses and my fellow-patients. I ran my hands over my body and with some surprise found that I was in no way disabled, except for the stiffness down my right side.

So I tried to get out of bed, thinking about my suitcase at the end of it. A nurse encouraged me to take a few steps across the floor, and in my wide knee-pants and great white smock, I got all the way over to my suitcase without any difficulty at all.

Astonishingly I could walk, almost as much as I could have wished. I got out my dressing-gown, slippers, socks and toilet articles, and after a brief spell of thought sitting on my bed, I walked, carefully, but with relatively steady steps out to the communal bathroom the nurse had told me was in the passage.

I was in the old part of the hospital, built almost a hundred years ago. The rooms were large and the corridors wide and endless, high-ceilinged and no doubt rather impractical. The bathroom was small and had two tiny compartments with basins and mirrors.

I shut myself into one of them. I washed and tidied myself up as best I could. That felt good. But one thing I dared not do – look at my undressed body in the mirror. I put on the great white smock before I started fixing my face and needed the mirror. I couldn't bear to look at myself as the invalid I was. I pushed it all away from me, contenting myself with glancing hastily at my right side as I undressed and dressed. The white bandages hid my right side from navel to shoulder. A glimpse at a time was all I could take.

The doctor came later on that morning. Clearly there was nothing much to say about me. The doctor smiled, looked at the bandage and said everything was as it should be, then asked me how I was feeling.

'Fine,' I said. Because I was. Wasn't I? I said to myself, slightly hesitantly. Yes, I was.

I had been through an operation in which they had cut away an essential part of myself and the anxiety about that was now over. A kind of paralysing relief came over me. I was fine, as I had told the doctor.

Now I was drawn into the little collective of six women in the ward. My interest in other people began to surface. One of them was a cheerful plump woman of about fifty who had been admitted for a varicose vein operation. She had been operated on at the same time as I had. She was in great pain and found it difficult to get out of bed. But something quite different was occupying her mind.

26

At the routine examination before her operation, they had found a growth below her left breast, and she had been given the same explanation as I had. They wanted to open the breast and according to what that indicated, they would then operate again or not. She was waiting with intense excitement for her doctor to come. She stared at me and asked me if they had . . .

'Yes,' I said, 'they have taken off my breast.' Her eyes turned large and black. I felt the anguish that was ravaging her. But then her doctor came to see her and told her, almost in passing, that no, the tumour was benign and her breast was saved. There would be no second operation.

There was one consonant's difference between her name and mine, and we had both been operated on at more or less exactly the same time. It turned out that a sister had muddled us up on the telephone, and given the wrong information to the families who had called. My brother was told that I hadn't needed a mastectomy, and her family that her breast had had to be removed.

We looked at each other, we two, and smiled, she as happily as anyone could be, and at the same with a genuine solidarity I prized beyond everything. I smiled back with all my heart. It was good to have a person nearby who had escaped.

I was soon to find out that not many people here had escaped. I was also to find out that my case was minor in comparison with my fellow patients'. Yes, in comparison with so many people I was to come into contact with in the corridors and departments all over the hospital.

The doctors said almost absent-mindedly that removing a breast and part of the lymph glands was no major surgical operation. It was 'uncomplicated'. At first I was relieved to hear this expert opinion, and in the wards I was to become close to women who had had far more serious surgery.

The magic circle threw a ring of fire round us in Ward 23. I would never have thought six totally strange women, their ages ranging from fifty to over eighty, all rather miserable and helpless, would be able to live together and feel such a natural closeness to each other. But that's what it was like.

Here our bodies were constantly tended. Constant care, day and night, from nurses and ward sisters, and the women who cleaned. Everything was done with discretion. But the bald truth was that our bodies were in a wretched state. Our most intimate weaknesses and human needs seemed to be highlighted by the physical proximity of the six of us in that little ward, which was indeed old-fashionedly high-ceilinged, but literally crammed with six beds and six bedside lockers. You could put up screens, but not everything can be concealed behind a screen.

All six of us probably each had our own private tragedy, which naturally enough, there was little room for. But there was also so much life in this small group of women – and great humour, occasionally really pungent humour.

A pretty, graceful little creature from Bergen delighted me one night, for instance. She had severe pains in her back, which were especially bad at night. In the daytime she was the light of our crippled little world, as she elegantly and playfully walked through the room in her red dressing-gown, her white-haired well-tended head held almost defiantly high, always obliging and helpful. The pain she suffered had left its mark on her lively face, but she was a strong little creature.

The nights were worst for her. One night she called to the sister for help, her pain critical. That was when I heard this well brought-up Bergen voice say: 'Give me a Holland's!'

The nurse, for they were mostly assistant nurses on duty at night, was a young girl from somewhere up along the west coast and was probably not particularly well acquainted with the multifold niceties of the world of alcohol. She didn't really catch what the lady was asking for. Then I heard again our little lady from Bergen say calmly, almost sharply, with a humorous undertone:

'Give me a Holland's Gin, I said!'

The pain in our bodies dominates us completely as it reaches a certain pitch. I had experienced very little physical pain in my life, because I had so very seldom been ill. For the first time, I came close to this part of life. It perhaps alters one's perspective.

For me, anyhow, those five days in Ward 23 were fundamental, a confrontation with obvious truisms, one could say, but which we *can* keep at arm's length for long spells of our lives. This business that the human body – our own – is something monstrously fragile, full of obstinate drive, indeed, but born to perish.

We are mortal. Those are words we say. And we probably say them constantly, in numerous automatic remarks throughout life.

But the way in which our western Christian civilization has developed, death today has become something we hide away. People from other cultures may see this as a sign that we are *obsessed with death*: that we have an hysterical and panic-stricken attitude towards death. I don't know. But the situation is probably that as long as one is young or healthy, the body's fragility, the misery of life and death, are things that concern only *others*.

I myself have behaved approximately like that. But direct contact with the stark reality of the hospital for those few days was a watershed.

I have no desire to keep it secret. There we were, six women, each in her own way shutting out the world in an all-absorbing fight against her own misery. It is like visiting the forecourt of the Kingdom of Death.

A remarkable expression that, perhaps – 'the Kingdom of Death', but as so little is ever said about such things today, we have very few words to draw on. Many people are afraid of 'big words'. They want to use words from the old books, from the days when people lived so much closer to death. Words like the Greeks' 'dark Hades', for instance. Or Dante's 'limbo, the forecourt of the Kingdom of Death'.

Nevertheless, one does feel 'the little words' – our chattering daily language – are inadequate. They flatten the soul, so that one feels spiritual as well as physical need.

Over this period of time my thoughts have often gone to Henrik Wergeland.

The remarkable thing about Wergeland is that he is eternally the poet who died young. He is perhaps no longer read by adults today. These days, youthful death probably causes nothing but sensitive shudders. But my thoughts have gone to Wergeland so often because this lover and master of words has said *it* in Norwegian, what in the Norwegian of today, we hardly dare let pass our lips.

Just listen to him from his sick-bed in the hospital in Christiania:

Is it ice rippling in my breast . . . ?
and those stabs of fire . . . ?
Let Death call it his victory.
It is my spring in heaven,
its dawning spring . . .
soon cold, soon hot,
my blessed April.

And the way in which he cries out:

Nought but Death will bring me reprieve

And listen to him, in all his wretchedness creating this poetry that could leave no heart cold, even in these petrified wordless days of ours:

Oh Spring! Spring! save me!
None has loved thee more tenderly than I.

I felt very strongly that only such 'big words' can help redeem what happens to you in the forecourt of death. But you can't lie reading Wergeland aloud in a hospital ward in Norway in this year of Our Lord, 1983, for visitors, relatives or friends might well regard you with some anxiety if you cried out 'Oh, Spring! Spring! save me!'

So there you are with your misery, side by side with the others. Objective medical expressions aren't really much help when it comes to using them yourself. The technical expressions you gradually learn in hospital are probably highly necessary for doctors and nurses surrounded day and night by our – i.e. 'other

31

people's' miseries. But we, the patients, cannot regard ourselves as patients!

So you have to try. Try not to be afraid of the big words, not to be so afraid of being private. You have to take the words you have, take them by the hand, as if they were small children, and lead them through this forecourt of death, this most ordinary of ordinary places in society today, but round which is a magic circle of burning silence.

A woman of about my own age was in the bed on my right. In all her behaviour, she gave the impression that she was not one of those who thought life, society, least of all the world owed *her* anything special. But one could see quite easily from her visiting family that for *them* she had a natural central place. The strength in that closed circle was as striking as the anonymity in the world outside.

She was no further away from me than that I could stretch out my hand and touch her. They had indeed put up a screen between us – a slight consolation to both of us. But she nevertheless must have taken part in my uneasy first night in the ward and I was to follow the course of her illness.

Never with distaste though. At first I was rather shaken by the extent of the scars her body was burdened with. But gradually that, too, became natural. I followed her struggles and victories when it came to making her shattered body function again, as if I had known her all my life.

There were two rows of beds in the ward, three beds in each row. In the row opposite was a woman who must have been about seventy. She had also been through the incredible craftsmanship of modern surgery, and as far as I could make out, several times in recent years.

She became the ward's source of experience, as people came and went. I noticed she had practically every kind of problem – lying in bed, sitting in bed, lying on one side, getting out of bed . . . for she *had* to do that. Doctors, nurses and physiotherapists all drove her on – out of bed and walk!

The toil of all this showed in her face, whether the days were hard or the nights sleepless. Getting her digestive system, blood vessels, muscles – yes, most parts of the body – functioning again was not easy. I noticed she often felt helpless, wretched. And how many times did I meet those steady, dark, despairing – but also determined – eyes of hers, as we lay in our beds opposite each other?

But she also had her victories, incredible and dearly-bought, such as when she managed to walk, with the physiotherapist's help, both up and down the long corridor outside the ward.

On my left was a woman well into her eighties. She had originally come from the north, and brought a breeze of the ocean and broad landscapes into the ward. It was hard to believe she was over eighty. But that's what she told us, fixing me with a challenging look. She had had one leg amputated below the knee a few years ago, and now she had had the other leg off. Her prothesis, the artificial leg replacing the first amputated leg, was propped up against the wall beside her bed.

Perhaps this all sounds rather macabre. Far from it. My neighbour was a source of life, humour and culture. And will-power. She was the youngest of us all, and she had an apparently boundless interest in everyone around her.

She was as industrious as an ant. She practised all day, with and without help, at getting out of bed into the wheelchair, out of the wheelchair back on to the bed. These training sessions were carried out with a joy that infected me, so the two of us almost regarded them as athletic achievements we might even take a bet on.

She was a delightful person, in both senses of the word. Her lively, upright figure, abundant white hair she coquettishly tended so well, the stern but at the same time gentle face with its open generous smile – they all made her an excellent neighbour. She was miserable, as we all were, of course, both legs gone from under her, and the struggle to overcome this, physically and 'administratively', was not easy in the Norwegian welfare state, which does not seem to be able to afford to give 'priority' to people as old as her.

When the conversation turned to that side of her problems, her eyes darkened into something rather like desperation. But she had other problems as well, such as, for instance, what she herself called 'my phantom pains' – pains in the recently amputated leg, which turned her nights into nightmares.

Twenty-four hours flows quietly by in a hospital ward, from morning to evening, with its definite rhythms of food and care, from evening to morning, with its minor and major dramas.

I slept a great deal. I read quite a lot. And I walked up and down the corridors, where I saw other sick people, other doctors, other nurses. My 'case' was clearly uncomplicated. That was the impression I got from what I saw, which often appeared much more dramatic.

After a few days, the time came for a 'major round'. A whole troop came into the ward, led by a middle-aged, loud-voiced and very energetic doctor. Behind him I caught a glimpse of the doctor who had operated on me, and behind him the nurses ranked in their hierarchy. The troop eventually arrived at my bed and the booming doctor proclaimed in a loud voice that I 'should realize' that the decision to remove my right breast had been taken after some considerable deliberations between a 'number of doctors'.

I stared numbly at him. Perhaps the man was trying to be kindly, but I was not prepared for this dramatic proclamation. What did he really mean? Had there been any chance of *not* removing my breast? I felt paralyzed.

I am far beyond the age when you find it difficult to talk, and all my life I have been in a profession that involves asking people things. But not a word passed my lips. I didn't know what to say. Perhaps I was looking at this loud-voiced doctor with a certain arrogance, because I had a vague feeling he was trying to start up a controversy with me, or something of the sort.

Why? I felt I was sinking through the bed. After declaring in the same booming voice that everything was going well and quite normally, the doctor marched off at the head of his troop to the next bed. After they had left the room, I realized I must contact the surgeon who had operated on me as soon as possible and extract some explanation of what had

35

been done to me and how I really was. This feeling that my 'case' was uncomplicated was perhaps pure illusion?

When I asked the ward sister, she said I had a 'fabulous' incision. Everything was fine. But she added: 'Have you looked for youself?'

I hadn't. I went into the bathroom every morning and evening, but I hadn't dared look in the mirror. You should, the ward sister said. As soon as possible, she thought. She no doubt knew what she was talking about as she nudged me in the direction of the mirror.

One day, I plucked up the courage. It was a difficult moment, I have to admit. Afterwards, I felt closer than ever to my fellow-patients in Ward 23, and as far as that was concerned, also all the other patients I met in corridors or caught harrowing glimpses of in the other wards.

We sick people. We carved up and maltreated human bodies of all ages and sexes, who found ourselves here, we all belonged together in my mind. Everyone else was 'out there', whether doctors, nurses or visitors.

We were *normal people*, they were *abnormal.*

The huge bustling medical apparatus that was functioning all round us was overwhelming. Everything that could be done, that *was* done, to the human body, this incredible modern medical machinery that carved people up and sewed them back together again, bringing them back to life – it was fundamentally unbelievable.

But *we sick people*, we were perfectly believable. We were a world of our own. We were naked humanity in extreme need, instinctively seeking each other out, while the doctors, nurses and visitors were all a distant and alien world.

I had felt I was stepping into a magic circle the first day I came into contact with this hospital. Now I felt I had arrived at the very centre of that circle.

It was at the same time both pleasingly safe and frightening. I felt solidarity with 'ordinary' sick people, and at the same time felt an uncontrollable desire to get away from it all, a longing to be able to get out of bed and run out of the hospital, out and back to the life I had put behind me that eternity of a few days ago.

Ward 23 was an acute surgical department, so no one stayed there very long. The whole idea was to get people out of bed and out of hospital as soon as possible. There were rows of new patients waiting for a bed.

Our plump cheerful fifty-year-old with varicose veins was the first to abandon us, excited and pleased. Then the neighbour on my right was launched on to her feet and left us, full of faith that things would be all right in her totally changed insides. Once they had gone new patients came.

One afternoon, the door opened and a bed came rolling in. Behind the three foot high white 'tent' I caught a glimpse of a stern, thin young woman. It turned out that her right leg was on a tall frame, covered with a sheet.

It was an articulate arrival. She never stopped talking, loud and clear, too, though it was difficult for the rest of us to catch the thread of her strong north-Trondheim dialect. In my mind, I baptized this young woman 'An-Magritt', from Falkberget's *Bread of Night*.

We gradually realized this young lady was not going to take anything lying down in silence. From the fragments we could make out, it appeared she was not going 'to put up with any old thing' from these doctors, these nurses. She was not going to stay 'longer than a day'. And why didn't someone come and 'examine her' anyhow? The torrent of words continued in an avalanche over by the door. My seventy-year-old fellow-patient opposite sent me a profoundly questioning look and pursed her lips.

After a while, 'An-Magritt' was moved alongside me. I tried a bit of light conversation. She stared acidly at me, but then gradually agreed to answer my questions. And she calmed down relatively soon.

Later that day, someone did come and examine her. Even I stiffened as I lay there in bed beside her. She had a great open wound on her right leg. It looked shattering to me, red and glaring, the size of half a loaf. Doctors and nurses flocking round her, however, were in their seventh heaven – a marvellous wound! and An-Magritt was also basically pleased with all the attention her incision was receiving.

Overt pain is relatively unknown in medicine today, for they have so many means of suppressing it that it is no longer a problem. I have experienced this myself. At no time has physical pain been an obtrusive problem for me, despite the fact they had cut deeply into me. This makes an operation just slightly unreal. And it was probably much the same for An-Magritt. She was now some kind of contented spectator of her own wounded leg.

But nevertheless . . . there is more to the human mind that one thinks, and An-Magritt's entrance into

38

the ward like a spitting wild-cat was evidence enough of that.

It was a reaction to anguish in a young, healthy and courageous little person. There was something liberating about her forceful assault. Most of us in the ward were older – anyhow, mature women. We also had our anxieties, some perhaps greater than hers. But we were probably more resigned, and also perhaps had more experience of the many blows and sorrows of life.

The nurses' reactions to An-Magritt's crackling arrival was interesting to observe. They took it quite professionally. Her torrent of words was utterly wasted on them. They did what they had to do to her and for her, ignoring the words lashing round the room. The rest of us were more agitated. But I don't think I am wrong when I say I think some kind of patient tenderness descended on us.

We had been sent something like a little wild flower and fundamentally it felt rather liberating to have someone in the ward who was simply not patient.

Of the whole complex medical staff of a hospital, naturally the nurses and assistant nurses were those we had most contact with. This was a totally new world to me, as I had so seldom been ill in my life. An impressive world, deep down, based on *care*.

It is a remarkable experience to be surrounded day and night by such care. Otherwise there is so little left of that kind of human feeling in our society that it is easy to imagine a hospital would also of necessity be cold and alien. But, no.

Here you find a group of people who have *chosen*

care. Of course, there is something deeply professional about it all, and I don't think either nurses or assistant nurses could go round truly suffering for all us patients. But I found it not *just* professional – for the care they gave us really was of a living kind. I confess that I myself would never have had the strength to choose such a profession. Gradually, as I observed nurses of all kinds with whom I came into contact, men as well as women, I came to the conclusion that such a profession could not *only* be a profession, but must in some way or other also be a vocation.

I am not so sure that doctors need necessarily feel any vocation, some kind of caring vocation, I mean. They are no doubt able to become absorbed in their subject, without much consideration for the person the patient also is. They *can* cut themselves off, I should say, in relation to the unfortunate creature in front of them.

But nurses can't do that. That is the only thing they can't do, and I have to say that however grateful I am to the doctors for saving me with their operations and treatments, it is the nurses who have my profound admiration.

For as your own condition gradually becomes less obtrusive, you begin to look around. You notice a night sister, with the patience of an angel, caring for, in the primary meaning of the word, a despairing fellow-patient's most intimate torments.

I have many memories of such nights. Nurses quietly talking, helping, arranging and calming – anonymous people, whose faces you often never see again. What is it that attracts young people to such a profession? I don't know. But I know it is something profoundly admirable.

It is also the nurses who take over when something more dramatic happens. A doctor may come in, perhaps decisively do something necessary. But the doctor disappears. It is the nurses who arrange everything else, including coping with a drama within the four walls of a ward with perhaps six or seven people lying there in a state of tension.

We experienced something of this kind in Ward 23 one day. A woman in her fifties, I should think, was pushed in and placed by the door. She was lying quite still. After an hour or so, however, she started whimpering, quite quietly at first, but then more and more loudly.

My seventy-year-old fellow-patient alongside her asked her something, and rang for Sister. Before she came, the woman's whimpering had become loud cries. She had unbearable pains in both legs, which later turned out to be a quite dramatic case of some kind of frostbite. In a very short while, the ward was transformed into a kind of emergency post, with Sister directing. A screen was brought in, several nurses tried to test the woman's reaction to touch, where the pain was and in what way it was developing. A doctor came, silently examined the woman and said that something would have to be done immediately. The preparation for what turned out to be an operation began.

All this was in the evening, the room dark and quiet, the woman's loud, agonized cries filling our little room with vague anguish, the nurses keeping everything under control.

We were all lying as quietly as frightened mice, each one in her own bed. But I think it highly probable that one of us *could* have been seized with active panic, if it hadn't been for the constant steadiness and calm of the nurses. In the course of an hour or two, the woman was taken out, and we understood it might be a matter of amputation. She left a vast silence behind her in the room.

Chapter Two

Admission to Ullevål Hospital had meant leaving this world, and during the six days and nights I was there another world appeared.

The magic circle that I had at first found frightening, later gradually came to seem almost secure. Time seemed to cease to exist there. Days and nights became eternities and brief glimpses. There was no 'before' – the shock had put everything into a grey area behind me. 'After' did not arise. I lived in a constant state of the present.

Meeting other patients in a worse state than myself probably helped strengthen this phenomenon. A kind of humility descended on me.

Gradually you noticed your strength, both physical and spiritual, coming back. I ate well. I slept well. I read a great deal, with much pleasure. In a strange way, I was quite happy. My surroundings gave me a sense of relief. I was alive.

Then when after only four days the doctors

started talking about discharging me and sending me home, I was panic-stricken. I spent six days altogether in hospital. But even when given two days to get used to the idea of going home, I looked forward to my departure with almost comical bewilderment.

This was mainly because I knew nothing about my own condition. I could feel the whole of my right side was stiff, and I told myself there might be problems managing on my own. But the efforts of close friends, family and acquaintances to help in practical terms and also encourage me, on the whole resolved most of that. I was also given a home-help to cope with shopping and other pressing matters.

But what about my own position? I had no idea.

My knowledge of cancer was what I suppose might be called abnormally limited. I found that most in my circle of friends knew far more than I did about current problems in relation to cancer in general and breast cancer in particular. I imagine the doctors thought I had a 'normal' knowledge of the subject, as I was in a position to ask about what was on my mind. But I really didn't know what to ask about.

Gradually, I assembled a number of questions I had planned to put to the surgeon who had operated on me. But in a modern hospital, there is no one you can call 'your doctor'. During the six days I had been at Ullevål, I dealt with four different doctors. In all my relations with the hospital and the various treatments I went through over a period of two months, I must have been in contact with ten or twelve different doctors.

Before my departure from the surgical unit, however, I had decided to talk to the doctor who had done the operation, at whatever cost. So I asked the ward sister, and other nurses with obvious authority, whether they could get the message to him to say 'I must talk to him' before I left. And I did talk to him.

That day, just as he had been on earlier occasions, he was exceptionally kind, speaking objectively in a quiet voice, and naturally humane, if also perhaps slightly distant.

He said that 'we have no indications' that the cancer had spread. According to my reading, I knew this meant that it was 'secondary metastases' that they had 'no indications of'. But the doctor added that it was a disease over which they had little control or grasp of, meaning I should have no illusions. But my lungs were not affected. That was always something, I thought.

'You have a good chance of total recovery,' the doctor said in a quiet, neutral voice. He explained that two days after I had been discharged from the surgical unit, I would be having one last treatment with chemotherapy. I had already had one dose in connection with the operation. A week later, the stitches would be removed. When I went to the surgical clinic for that, they would then have the final results of the operation. Not until then would they know whether the cancer had spread into the lymph glands, and whether radium treatment would eventually be necessary.

I understood this to mean that the chances of that were small. Or rather, I was so pleased that apparently neither my lungs nor any other organs were affected, and I was so ignorant, I simply came to the conclusion that after the last chemotherapy dose it would all be over.

*   *   *

In the afternoon, six days after the operation, I once again climbed the stairs to my apartment in Vika in Oslo. It was the same apartment block, the same stairs, the same home. But I was probably a different person.

It is difficult to describe this. I know there are huge inarticulate areas within people, areas where primary emotions rule, where experiences that are intuitive as opposed to reasoned can be unusually insistent, and how deeply buried traces of our lives can come to the surface.

The doctor who told me that from a surgical point of view a mastectomy is quite uncomplicated is undoubtedly right. Nevertheless, deep down I felt an elementary rebellion, beyond all logic and reason. When the first shocked fear had dispersed, and I found myself at home in my own bed, in my own room, among my own possessions, *grief* welled up in me, grief for a part of me that had gone.

Every day, I plucked up my courage and looked at myself in the mirror in the bathroom or in my bedroom. It was shattering.

It was an emotion beyond reason, which with automatically recurring words kept assuring the inarticulate part of me that my right breast was not an organ necessary for life, as were my lungs, for instance, or my heart.

Nevertheless, I found myself bursting into completely motiveless tears, overcome by some inner tumult. I called it grief, because I had no other word for these tears that poured down, suddenly and from depths I felt were an extremely real part of myself.

Several doctors I was in contact with took the initiative and talked to me about this. Apart from the

46

lack of surgical complications, which they so sooth-
ingly emphasized, they talked – in particularly friendly
terms – about the psychological complications I would
have to cope with. I listened to them without saying a
word.

I naturally received the logic they were trying to
get over to me with gratitude. I felt they wished me
well. But *I* knew with all my emotional life that I had
lost something very important. A breast is for a
woman not just a 'symbol of femininity', as I saw it
described in a book on cancer, nor simply a mammary
gland. I can live without 'symbols' and am past the age
of motherhood. But a breast is also a very important
part of emotional life. If it is removed, the incision
goes directly into that emotional life, into what is the
most elementary psychic and erotic part of you.

I felt it would lead to no good at all to deny this. I
had to look it in the eye, and live through it. So I said
not a word to the doctor's remarks.

The best support I had was from a woman
doctor. She looked very prosaically at me and said I
would have to reckon on it getting worse before it got
better. I think she had an instinctive understanding of
what I had been through. Anyhow, I liked her down-
to-earth realism, and when one day she said quite
objectively that 'one day you'll have got used to it',
then I knew as if in a vision that she was right.

I knew enough about myself and perhaps about
human nature to know that there are no limits to what
we can get used to. Those brief, unsentimental, but
nevertheless very personal comments from that
woman doctor did me good.

So I admitted relatively quickly that I would have
to live through the vale of tears I was sunk in, until

47

life-force itself slowly hauled me out into the daylight and *joie-de-vivre* again. I cried in the most surprising places and observed myself with a mixture of terror and attempts at self-realization.

I could burst into floods of tears in the open street if anyone showed me the slightest kindness. It was like being without your skin, like being flayed. I was terrified of my tendency to become furiously angry or to be 'seduced' by people's kindness. With great difficulty, I managed to accept myself in this over-emotional state. You have to live through it, I said to myself. Without shutting yourself in.

At the same time, I clung to the more 'reasonable' side of myself. This new disability of mine, for instance. The whole of my right side was stiff, as I mentioned before. I had a great long wound that ran across the right side of my breast and under my armpit. I can't say I had much pain, as long as I didn't move that arm or my body too much. But I noticed that I was walking with my arm kept continuously bent, as if in some kind of defensive position. It hurt to lift my arm, and I was constantly afraid I would bump into someone or someone would bump into me.

A friend I have known for forty years and whose subject is the functions of the body told me categorically to go to a physiotherapist and exercise that arm. Nor did she give in. She had to keep calling me for a whole day on the telephone before I took the plunge and contacted a physiotherapist in my own street.

I telephoned for an appointment, feeling that the 'sensible' part of me was in charge. For the first time since I had left the doctor's surgery having been told that I may have cancer, I was functioning actively. I was overcome with tremendous energy. Now I would not give up until I had arranged an appointment with the physiotherapist, and I was given one at once, for the very next day.

But by then some of that energy had disappeared. The skin-less me, with all its anxiety and perpetual tiredness, had appeared again.

I screwed myself up to go for that appointment. I was bathed in sweat, my mouth dry, and even rather frightened of showing my carved-up torso. But I managed to get myself on to the physiotherapist's couch in a state of semi-undress. And I probably lay down so that I couldn't see her face when she looked me over.

The physiotherapist turned out to be an extremely peaceable person, under any circumstances. She started her treatment of the arm and shoulder as if it were the most natural thing in the world, as I lay there with my gigantic scar. I came out of the Institute that day with a sense of relief. So something could be done! I could do something! I had been given some light exercises to do at home and I set about them with furious energy. This was something *outside* that magic circle of the hospital, and it did me good.

Friends and acquaintances paid warm attention to me. But I avoided them. I couldn't cope with people. I became indescribably weary after a short time and felt a profound need to be by myself.

This was difficult to describe, and neither did I try to. I perhaps hurt friends who wished me nothing but well. But I had no surplus strength. On the other hand, I did turn to books, feeling a strong desire to read things that went into more depth, not simply entertainment or a pastime.

I hunted around in a bookshop down in the city, looking for a book or a theme that would respond to something indefinite I was fumbling after. I found several. A new long American biography of Karen Blixen. An equally long book by an Englishwoman on the history of Buddhism.

And then I began looking back into books I had read many times before. The French *Madame de Sevigne*, for instance, or Colette, and a big book I had had on my bookshelves for a long time without reading it – a learned treatise on the Greek historian and travel writer, Herodotus's view of the world outside Hellas – feeling an intense joy at being able to become engrossed in questions and themes that had absorbed me all my life.

It was in connection with this that my thoughts suddenly touched on an ancient legend I had been absorbed by, the legend of the Amazons, a (mysterious?) group of people whom, among many others, both Homer and Herodotus mention. Homer called them *Antianeria*, which according to the experts is a sufficiently ambiguous expression that it can be translated as either 'men's equal' or 'men's enemy'.

As the Amazons were a mounted warrior tribe from a distant and, to the Greeks, unreal North outside the Hellenic world, they might possibly have been not only equal to the Greek warriors, but also their enemies. War was a matter of honour in those days.

Otherwise, Herodotus called them, perhaps more prosaically, *A-mazons*, which means 'without breasts'. The legend had it that they cut off their right breasts in their youth in order to be able to handle their bows and arrows more easily on horseback.

These Amazons appear constantly in the Greek heroic legends as part of the Hellenic wars and victories over the barbarians – in other words, everything not Greek. Great heroes such as Heracles, Theseus and Achilles have all fought legendary battles against Amazon queens such as Hippolyte, Antiope and Penthesilea.

The Amazon Queen Penthesilea, according to the legends, came to the assistance of the Trojan Hector at the battle of Troy. She fought hand-to-hand with Achilles, the great Greek hero, who killed her, only to discover at the moment of death that she was a woman. This scene has been made much of in Greek art, the legend running that the noble Achilles wept as the sword plunges into brave Penthesilea.

It is strange how your mind can centre on half-forgotten stories and impressions when you find yourself in a kind of border-country of the soul. Suddenly I remembered that I had seen Greek vase paintings portraying just that struggle between Achilles and Penthesilea. Why should I remember that *now*?

Because I – like Penthesilea – had had my right breast cut off? I smiled at myself.

Burying yourself in books is something that could be light-heartedly self-ironic and at the same time fascinating and rather pleasant. Greek art and literature, especially of the early Archaic period, is something that has interested me all my life. So I have quite a number of books on the subject, and several grandiose illustrated works. I buried myself for several days in these books, searching for those illustrations of Achilles and Penthesilea I could only just remember. It was a feast.

This lavish fantasy-world left behind by the Greeks, with their strong faith and great art, is to me a constant source of humanity. I found several portrayals of the Amazons astonishingly beautiful for barbaric monsters.

There was, for instance, this vast painting from an early period, in which the fearsome, helmeted, super-warrior Achilles, his head bowed in grief, is carrying the dead warrior Queen Penthesilea over his shoulder, away from the battlefield.

These early Greek paintings tell you a great deal. A certain naïvety, a freedom from the psychological interpretations with which we are so burdened today, stamps these vigorous Greek legends. The Amazons clearly fascinated Greek men, not always innocently, I should say. They were often portrayed and described along the lines of barbaric monsters such as sea-serpents, man-eating oxen and wild lions living outside the 'civilized' walls of Hellenic cities. Barbarians to be civilized. But as I said before, there is something disarmingly naïve about this Greek openness.

The Amazons were possibly a constant night-mare to the Greeks – truly mysterious people, who were not only fought but also at the same time admired in the eternal play of life and death and society of the legends. But it is also possible there may have been a touch of reality behind the legends, a very distant reality, perhaps, and distorted by Greek ideology. But it is historically accepted that many different peoples outside the world of Greece, who were called barbarians, such as the Scythians in the

52

north or Asiatic groups in the east, had quite different life-styles from that of the Greeks.

So there may possibly have existed a people up in the northern outposts where the women were also warriors, and where the brutal Greek division between men who were warriors and women who were mothers did not exist. Historians of today have on the whole, both in archaeology and linguistics, reassessed the unambiguous enthusiasm for the unique 'civilizing' effect of Hellenic culture of many previous generations.

The possibility that civilizations existed in Asia and northwards into Europe, which the Hellenic forces simply crushed, but which were not necessarily any less 'civilized', has struck many people. Our day has a greater sense of the multiplicity in the history of mankind that previous generations had, and the Amazons have always been to me a riddle worthy of interest.

But what *was* this sickly over-sensitivity I was really seeking in this search for portrayals of the Amazons?

It was a game. A game of identity.

It is not easy to accept one's own body, reduced to its essential parts. I have, for instance, a portrait of myself, painted by my father when I was about six or seven years old. A thin childish body. I looked at it and said to myself: Is this how your life will end, coming full-circle – back to the thin child-body? It was a game with little joy in it, and I turned away from it.

The Amazons were much more interesting. That was pure fantasy, which could also take my thoughts into distant myths. In that way, I was suddenly neither an invalid nor necessarily condemned to death.

That was *happy* escape, which for periods of time could chase away the anguish, and considerably more radically than any tax authority with its poverty-stricken and complicated regulations was able to. I believe in escapism that is filled with joy. I truly believe it is a way in which we human beings can learn to live with realities that may appear to be unbearable.

For unpleasant realities are inescapable. I was indeed given a week's grace after being discharged from the hospital surgical unit. Two days later, I was back again for my dose of chemotherapy. I also had my physio-therapy session in my own street. But I was living under the great illusion that the worst was over.

Possibly, I had blocked out the realities, simply by not trying to find out more about what this cancer of mine really involved. I simply allowed myself to float along on events.

But a week after my discharge I was back at the hospital to have my stitches out. That turned out to be a mere bagatelle. Afterwards, I had a talk with one of the doctors and he was able to tell me the famous diagnosis on the basis of the results of the operation.

During the operation they had removed ten lymph glands and in one of these, they had found a nodule, i.e. cancer symptoms. So the spread of it was a fact, if only of a relatively weak nature statistically.

Then I was told that the medical routine, when there were, as in my case, any signs of spreading, was that you had radium treatment. In addition, and as another boost for this routine, it turned out that the tumour in my right breast had been a large one.

My reaction to this was renewed anguish that

manifested itself in desperate attempts to find a way out. I asked the doctor whether this was really necessary! He replied that it was routine. At which I again asked if the routine were necessary!

He smiled gently and explained that I would be transferred to a doctor in the Radiotherapy Department, who would explain to me anything of that kind I wished to know. What would *that* doctor say if I refused radium treatment? I asked, with assumed objectivity. The doctor replied that he would probably shake his head a little . . . but that he had made an appointment for me at the radiotherapy department for twelve days later and all I need do was to go there . . .

The doctor also told me that he had assisted at my operation. He had talked to me in the operating theatre, he said. I realized that I had asked him questions. I had wanted to know what they had done to me.

Did I remember any of this? the doctor asked me. I remembered absolutely nothing. 'No,' said the doctor. 'I thought that would be so, so I asked you whether we could talk about it later.'

I looked more closely at the man. He was relatively young, and he had also visited me while I was in the surgical unit. But I had no memory whatsoever of him in the operating theatre, nor the slightest recollection of any conversation with him. So here was that mystery of the anaesthetic and the operation again, in a much more obtrusive form.

I had twelve rather difficult days ahead of me until I had to go to the radiotherapy department at the hospital. My fear of radium treatment and my reluctance on the whole to accept it, overwhelmed me, and on top of that, there was this mystery of the anaesthetic. I often woke at night with nightmares.

These night fears were completely vague. I could neither put words nor shape to them, but they kept recurring, regularly every night, and several times during the night.

I had a vague indistinct sense of 'something' inside me being driven – that is what it felt like – towards the black wall that was the anaesthetic and the operation. It was as if something inside me were trying to get through that wall. Or perhaps it was something trying to get out of that darkness? It was all very indistinct, and at the same time impossible to escape.

I tried everyone I came into contact with, nurses, doctors, even my physiotherapist, and asked whether it were physically possible that eventually, with intense hard work, I could penetrate into a consciousness within myself that had 'memories' of the operation?

I must have expressed myself very badly, as no one seemed to understand what I was talking about. But this burning question occupied me for several months, less so later on, but always obtrusively. I felt – or thought I felt – that 'something' inside me had suffered a shock.

I imagined that the actual surgical intervention, by which I mean the operation on my breast, had been 'registered' by some of my nerves or other organs. I also imagined this 'something' inside me worked itself violently up to the surface while I was asleep, causing these vague sensations and, in the real sense of the word, primordial fears that woke me.

Was any of this possible? I asked. Could I 're-capture' awareness of what had happened to me during the operation? For I did know one thing – I could remember absolutely nothing whatsoever of the many hours I was under the anaesthetic. Those long hours were surrounded by a black wall. Did 'something' attempt to penetrate through that wall? Or was the conscious me trying to penetrate it? And in that case, was it at all possible?

I felt I was talking to a brick wall when I put such questions to doctors and academics. I had a feeling they thought either I was crazy, or that they might possibly have an answer, but I would not be able to take it. It was actually my physiotherapist who took the greatest interest in the matter. She told me about a friend of hers who had had to have a Caesarian operation, so gave birth under an anaesthetic. She had an intense feeling afterwards of having 'been cheated' of the birth.

As the physiotherapist remarked, this was not really comparable. I couldn't have any sense of having having been cheated by my operation, as I put it. But there *were* other people who had had remarkable feelings after an anaesthetic.

Someone will now say that this is all sheer speculation, and I have a feeling that many surgeons probably regarded it as that. I admit that I do have a tendency to think all the time, possibly too much. One should really have a greater capacity to abandon oneself to fate than I have. Many people I have talked to also regard anaesthetic as a happy chance to abandon oneself and let things happen painlessly. I should no doubt have learnt a little more about abandonment.

It is also regarded as a very 'female' quality, possibly acquired, and anyhow useful during many of the caprices of life. But it is clearly a quality I have too little of, so what they called 'speculations' continued to torment me.

One reason was also that all this was at its most obtrusive at night, taking the form of profound and unexpressed anguish. So my 'speculations' were also emotionally based.

It was suggested that I should take Valium, or sleeping tablets, and generally try to suppress my anxieties with available aids. I had little desire to do this. On the contrary, I dearly wished not to suppress anything, anyhow as long as I could bear it, and instead attempt to explore this anguish.

One is what one is. If I were someone with what to others seemed an exaggerated awareness, then it was no solution for me to allay this urge with drugs. My anguish might then possibly grow even greater.

The same physiotherapist said something one day that put me on the track. While she was treating my arm, she said rather casually that maybe it wasn't all that strange, as I was perhaps a person who had difficulty accepting anything being done to me, except by myself, so to speak.

She said it very nicely, not as a comment on my personality. But it was a new key for me. Suddenly I saw myself as the exceptionally obstinate person I was.

Oh, that went a long way back! As far back into my childhood as I can remember. Over the years, I have probably grown milder, a little more tolerant. But the same inflexible hostility to being forced, inflicted or imposed on with anything I had not accepted myself, or even sought for, is still there in my whole personality. And this time I had been brutally 'imposed on', after having first been put right out of

58

the picture with an anaesthetic. As this had been done to me, and in addition an essential part of my body taken away, perhaps it was not all that remarkable that I was having nightmares.

Rather slowly, I began to feel that my search for physical answers as to the possible chances of 're-capturing' my operation were perhaps not all that important. Maybe it was more important to admit to oneself what one was, and so find a way to adapt oneself to circumstances.

On the Monday after Palm Sunday, at 9.30 in the morning, I went to Ulleval Hospital for my appointment at the Radiology Department – or the 'Radio-therapy Section', as the department is called.

So I had to find my way into yet another world: following the esoteric notices – *Radiotherapy, Isotope, Cobalt Unit* – to the place in question, a small group of chairs and a table where many other people were also waiting; glancing at more notices containing what were to me barbaric words such as 'nuclear medicine'; sitting down with the others and waiting, where one of those extremely friendly, authoritative nurses was in charge like a hen seeing to her clutch of chicks.

At this point – after twelve days of reflection and somewhat confusing 'consultations' with doctors and other informed people – I had given up all thoughts of refusing radium treatment. I had admitted the stupidity of my resistance, but I was depressed.

I was a 'free' patient, I know. I was not going into something quite unknown, as with the operation. There was no plastic strap round my wrist, as I had had for the operation. That same morning, I had cleared up a huge heap of papers dealing with my illness and had found that small identity band; a small strip of paper inside a narrow plastic strip, on which was typed my date of birth and another number which was no doubt my patient-number – 16 digits in all. That was me. But my name and address were also there. Order in all things.

I had cut that plastic strap off as soon as I reached home with a feeling of having got free . . . No such number this time, but here I was again, sitting waiting, for another round of something about which I knew nothing.

The consultant in the radiotherapy department was also a pleasant man. He took his time. First he described my case – the operation during which the breast and lymph glands had been removed and how they had found a 'secondary' in one of the glands.

He apologized for the expression 'daughter-tumour', which is the ordinary Norwegian expression for a secondary metastasis. I had not reacted. He looked relieved. I thought to myself that the equal rights campaign has certainly come a long way in Norway, but at that particular moment I didn't care whether they called it a 'daughter-tumour' or a 'son-tumour'.

The doctor asked me whether I knew what cancer was, to which I said no. He gave me a brief and clear introduction to the disease. I took special note of the fact that a cancer tumour is an over-production of one's own cells, a growth that destroys normal tissue.

The doctor said that they had no 'positive' grounds for thinking any of the cancer remained after the operation. Nevertheless, there was always a certain risk of that. They had already tried to counteract that risk by giving me chemotherapy during the operation and another dose seven days later. In addition to this, they now wanted me to have radium treatment.

This would be given close to the areas where the surgeon had operated, and as a safety measure in some adjacent areas. The effect of the radium was to destroy the cells' ability to divide, thus preventing development of cancer cells. The treatment would last about five weeks, with radiotherapy each weekday.

Five weeks! Every day! It was going to be much worse than I had imagined. But I felt resignation descending on me.

The doctor said that I might find I had a sore throat after a few weeks, or my skin might feel sore. Some people became tired and listless, he said. But otherwise it was all totally painless. And, as he had said, it was a safety measure.

At this time, I was beginning to look in my 'cancer book' in earnest, as it was obvious that I was by no means as in the clear as I had thought. I found out that I had a fifty per cent chance of not having a recurrence within the next five years. But at the same time, there was also a fifty per cent chance of so-called secondaries lying latent somewhere in my body and breaking out one day.

Now it was a matter of simply giving my body whatever chances were available. Radium treatment was one of those chances. I gave in with some nervousness, but I was determined to make the best of it. The consultant said that if I wished, I could leave the treatment until after Easter, in other words, to be given ten days grace.

I seized this with enthusiasm. To have ten days without any treatment struck me as happiness.

Those ten days became a kind of strangely stolen freedom. Use these days, I said to myself. I tried to create peace within me, by reading things I enjoyed, by eating and drinking things I liked, and going on outings to Bygdøy, a place I had known since I was a child and which I love. My physiotherapist was also away on her Easter holidays at this time, so I had the whole day at my disposal.

The trips to Bygdøy were wonderful. Spring was late that year, so the snow still lay in patches in the Kongskogen woods. It was that lovely time of transition between winter and spring, when the countryside is on the point of taking off. Everything is still, not a green blade of grass yet to be seen, the bare silhouettes of the trees forming the most delicate network of subdued nuances of colour against a light grey sky, or a blue spring sky.

I had many wonderful experiences, such as in the forest of young birches out at Paradise Bay, which each day produced a different delicate silhouette against a constantly changing sky; one day the closely clustered white young trunks outlined against a transparent blue sky, the next day shining phosphorescently against a dark grey sky. One day the tree trunks were immobile, the next day swaying in the wind.

And Oslo fjord beyond might one day be perfectly calm, reflecting an old boat-house on a point in the water of the fjord, a replica of itself so clear and regular that it was difficult to distinguish between the boat-house and the reflection in the water; days like those, when even the gulls bobbing on the water were reflected in the fjord, a fantasy landscape so quiet, people could be heard talking in houses far away.

Inside the Kongskogen woods, the first humble buds of blue anemones had appeared, curling up towards the light from beneath their thick rubber-like leaves. Everything was rustling and rippling. We waded through slush and mud in the woods, listening to the birds singing at the tops of their spring voices, and taking in the smell of earth, of dead leaves, of pine trees and the sea.

I could walk like that for hours, my body functioning reasonably well, although my right side was still rather stiff, taking deep draughts of the early spring air and the countryside, and feeling how they banished my anguish and worries with an ease that says a great deal about how dependent human beings are on nature for their spiritual health.

In my wanderings round bookshops in central Oslo, I had found a book that had caught my interest, a book about Buddhism written by the English 'novelist, social-historian and expert on Asia, Nancy Wilson Ross.' That was how she was described on the jacket. I had never heard of her before.

The religions of Asia were not subjects I had gone into very much. I would even say that in my work as a journalist, with its obviously Asian subjects such as China and the Vietnam war, I had quite consciously kept such questions at an arm's length. The Middle East and Africa, the border countries between Islam, Christianity and the animistic religions, were areas that had seemed to fill my leisure time to an extent that Asian ideas had not impinged on me.

But the great thing about the world of books is

that in it one can always find new and interesting things. However long a human life is, it would never be long enough for the tremendous wealth lying hidden in the world of books.

This book about Buddhism that I found on a shelf in a bookshop in the middle of Oslo was one of several that I happened to take down and look at. I leafed through it. I soon realized Nancy Wilson Ross's book was no militant Buddhist book of the more exalted and evangelical kind that can be found virtually all over Europe.

I do not like exalted evangelists whether Christian, Islamic, Buddhist or Marxist-Leninist. We have a great many of them these days, the bookshops overflowing with their near-hysterical pamphlets. But this was a 'serious' book, a thorough and intelligent account of the history of Buddhism and its different forms and expressions throughout the centuries, all over the world, including in the world of art. It became one of the books I stuffed into my plastic bag and took home to my apartment in Vika.

That Easter in 1983, over those ten days of oddly gained freedom, I read Nancy Wilson Ross's book. It was a great surprise to me. My ignorance of Buddhism was great. I discovered that Buddha was a human being, a man who had really lived six hundred years before Christ.

His historical life resembled to a great extent other religious founders, such as Jesus of Nazareth or Muhammad, such as Socrates, too, not to mention all the men and women in the world whom many regard as saints, and others regard as philosophers or artists, who over the ages have been obsessed by the tragic riddle of mankind.

There is a striking resemblance between all these men and women. Metaphysical or religious unrest obsesses their lives to such an extent that they become totally involved, in contrast to the numberless masses of the rest of us, who have had no time, or who have not made time for more than brief glimpses into such matters.

Neither will I hide the fact that this spring of 1983 was a brief glimpse into my life when such matters seemed urgent.

Death is man's dilemma. And my cancer had brought death, the reality that I myself was actually mortal, close to me. I must say that until then I had thought much like the French writer Colette, who says somewhere that death does not interest her, least of all her own death.

Not that my interest had really increased, but the question could no longer be ignored.

Buddha – or Siddhartha Gautama – as this man from a country near the Himalayas was called – in Nancy Wilson Ross's book turned out to be an astonishing person, almost like someone of my own time. In that respect, there was nothing particularly unusual in his fundamental unrest, a well-known aspect of all religions and all art. But the circumstances of his life, 2,500 years ago, were astonishingly close and familiar, if you extract the exotic details round the son of a king in a small kingdom in northern India, whose father worshipped him as the most valuable jewel in the world.

With a little imagination, we who today live in the small kingdom of Norway up towards the borders of the Arctic can all be regarded as royal children in a sheltered word of affluence.

What this young Gautama discovered when he made forbidden nightly excursions outside his sheltered world of wealth, beauty and security, was just what we all discover when the fundamental riddle and crises of life touch us.

Outside the palace's hanging gardens, he came across an *old* man, a *sick* man, and a *corpse* – in fact, death. It was a shattering revelation to him, that no one escapes old age, the sufferings of the body, or sorrow and loss apparently impossible to bear.

Gautama's reaction to this 'vision', if the legends about him are true, could be regarded as 'very modern'. He felt that life was *absurd*. Why should anyone wish to be born at all, not to mention give birth to a child, when in the end everything ends in loss, sorrow and suffering?

Buddha's approach is as old as man. All art from the dawn of time is about this, and naturally all religion. Buddha's solution to the anguish of life – or fear of death – was to go out on to the road as a beggar and seek out the wise men who could tell him what the meaning of life was. And so he ended up by creating a new religion.

The story of Siddhartha caught my imagination, most of all because Buddha did not pretend to be a God, nor even a 'son of God' or a 'prophet'.

He spent his life on this clarification, but he finally created a religion in which man was no special God-ordained creature, and in which he himself was no special divine messenger.

This aspect of Buddha meant that my interest in him simply increased with the reading of Nancy Wilson Ross's book. I felt strongly that Buddha's solutions were also 'modern', although his individual theories and methods interested me less. It was this fundamental conclusion of Buddha's that intrigued me – that man is an integral part of the universe and that it is his tragic need, with his feverish ego, to oppose this universal unity and solidarity that produces such an insistent sense of the absurdity of life.

Like most people, as long as I can remember, I have pondered on the riddle of life. I have had my fair share of untroubled happiness. It is not that. But I have never been indifferent to the 'riddle of life' or the 'tragedy of life'.

At the same time, I am an agnostic, specifically agnostic in relation to Christianity and other religions (there have been many over the centuries) that organize the world and the universe into hierarchical concentrations of power, with a God at the top as ruler, and Mankind (mostly Man) as the particularly loved apple of the ruler's eye.

I am probably not alone in this confusion in relation to religion. On the contrary, I notice it is a strong current in my day, a period of time which in so many ways has been forced into questioning religious beliefs, and political beliefs as well, for that matter. For me, it has been a slow and not particularly dramatic process over a period of forty years.

I grew up in an agnostic home, but not many church people would go so far as to call it a 'heathen' home. My mother was a parson's daughter, and that side of the family had strong roots in evangelism, and before that in Haugianism, a popular movement named after Hans Nilsen Hauge, and Ryfylke's popular religious movements on the west coast. But as a child, I remember my mother saying 'a pastor's child is the devil's child.'

She had certainly not been a 'child of the devil' in her life, far from it. But her generation, those who were young immediately after the first world war, went through the first wave of de-Christianization in Norway, and that particularly affected the children of church ministers.

As far as my father's family is concerned, my grandfather and grandmother on that side were Swedish 'guest-workers', and although neither was especially active in the worker's movement, they were probably a natural part of the currents dominating the Scandinavian working-class at the end of the last century and the beginning of this one, and agnosticism was part of that.

The point, however, is that I did *not* grow up in any aggressively anti-Christian environment. My maternal grandmother, a very important person in my life, was a great believer from Sand in Ryfylke and had moved to Kristiania as a young pastor's wife. I lived all my childhood with her untroubled air of pious and upright Christian faith around me, but at the same time, with my parents' definite if respectful lack of faith.

In puberty, I went through a conversion crisis that no doubt stemmed from opposition to my parents, but since I was about twenty Christianity has meant little to me. Today, you could say I am neutral towards it, but respect those who believe, provided their faith is not a pretext to persecute or suppress other people's faiths; and except that I have great appreciation for the original Christian writings, a dominating part of the cultural heritage of my own society.

Why am I talking about all this? Because I think my own example is fairly common in the Norway of the Eighties, and actually even more common in generations younger than my own.

A failing of the church and most involved Christians is to presume that this general mass of people, like myself, do not concern themselves at *all* with the riddle of life, that we are 'heathens' in the sense that we are rigid 'rationalists' and single-minded 'materialists'. I have never considered myself any of those, and I think I can say quite objectively that that is not the case.

I am agnostic, but do not reject religious feelings, to the extent that I honestly believe they are a profound need in all human beings. But what has troubled me about Christianity, increasingly over the years, is its pretentious attitude in the universe, on our own planet and towards mankind. It is an organization I find little backing for around me, or within myself.

Naturally this is primarily the old story of the church's portrayal of God as a kind or tyrannical (according to some) man – or 'Father', as they say, surrounded by the Son, and the Holy Ghost, who clearly also has to be categorized as some kind of male spirit. I am sure that these are meant as images, symbols if you like, but in all modesty, images and symbols that are meaningless to me. Neither is it any more meaningful or satisfactory to know that the church has elaborated on them for two thousand years.

Not that things would be much better if God were a kind or tyrannical woman – surrounded by the Daughter and a feminine Holy Ghost. It is the actual human-centering – in this case male – of the Divinity that is alien to me. I don't believe in it. I certainly admit, indeed am sure that in the past Christianity became an important humane life-form for European peoples in their time, for Norwegians as well. But that does not help.

Today, Christianity appears to be an empty shell, and its distinctive historical qualities still plough crudely on. There is little connection between this image and what science has managed to uncover and this distinctively man-centred world-order. The idea of a male god sitting somewhere out in the universe occupying himself particularly with human beings, I find a touchingly naïve image, similar to the ancient Greek Homer's depiction of the gods.

Just think how he saw the world! Just take his depiction of that vigorous Greek assembly of gods, every one of them taking a stand from one side or the other in the famous Trojan wars, for instance, and how all the gods placed themselves in a kind of heavenly grandstand and eagerly followed the great and bloody battles between Trojans and Achaeans on that tiny little battlefield outside the walls of Troy.

Today we can laugh at such an idea. It is at best touching, when one does not believe it. But it becomes rather frightening should someone insist that it is true. I have a slight feeling that Christianity is going much the same way, if in a much more sophisticated manner, and undoubtedly less bloody. But the churches obviously believe that their God is sitting somewhere in the universe and following with particular interest what mankind is up to on this tiny little planet.

* * *

70

For me this de-Christianization has been a long and relatively undramatic process. It has also happened within a strong and apparently secure current of my own day and in my own country. But then something very strange appears.

Death has no place here. It is hidden away. It is reduced to silence in our entire culture.

This is fundamentally a rather extraordinary development for our culture, in which for over two thousand years death has played such a dominating role – so much so that quite recently a man like India's Nehru, from a completely different culture, on his first meeting with Europe as a young man in his twenties, literally recoiled with loathing over what he felt was our society's 'obsession with death', particularly dramatically illustrated, he thought, in the realistic dead Christ he kept coming across everywhere.

And today, only sixty years later, death is denied to the extent that even the churches now seem to be concealing the twisted body of Christ, and instead bringing out a 'fourpence-off Jesus' beyond punishment and death and judgement, a totally cosy character. Even more striking, perhaps, is that one seems to be able to sense an underlying expectation that Social Services have banished death – indeed, that this is a human right the Ideal State aims at for us all, although it has perhaps not yet been successful for the particularly crippled individual, who under no circumstances is ever oneself, but someone else.

The result of this remarkable development in our society is that death has also been driven underground in each individual.

Death has become taboo, just as sexuality was previously. One can sense the same loathing of

71

anything 'animal' that the Christian world felt for so long for biological man.

Has death in our de-Christianized society been turned into the 'animal' in us? Naturally, it turned out in the Christian world that the biological animal in us could neither be got rid of nor suppressed, despite the long periods of time when they managed to warp it.

I think our de-Christianized society will discover that neither can death be suppressed, without society becoming warped and frightening. I ask myself: 'The aggressive anguish so typical of our time – yes, even the remarkable mixture of brutality and raw oversensitivity that is so evident – is it not the "illegalizing" of death in our midst that is the cause of it?'

In his last book, published a few months before his death in 1982, Father Hallvard Rieber-Mohn says:

'What is new in recent European and western civilization . . . is the mass-deviation from a handed-down religious interpretation of death. As a collective mental process, it totally lacks any parallel in the historically known past, and is consequently a "civilizational experiment" *with at the moment utterly incalculable effects and long-term mental consequences that today can hardly be imagined.*' My italics.

Father Rieber-Mohn was a person I felt an intuitive contact with, despite our different views of life, he a Catholic and I agnostic. The reasons were many, one of them being our common tie with a Latin and French world that neither for him nor for me entailed subjection, but seemed to be an enrichment, both in jest and seriously. So at this time I often felt sorrow over not being able to talk to a person like

72

Rieber-Mohn. In the chapter 'Death in the Middle Ages' in his book *Stone on Stone, Five looks at Sigrid Undset,* which turned out to be his last, he displays a deeper understanding of the new conditions of death in our de-Christianized world than anyone in our society, including most of our de-Christianized establishment.

I often felt in that spring of 1983 that there was no one I could talk to about these matters, because confusion reigned, surrounded by a secret taboo. The lack of a Rieber-Mohn at times seemed to be an ominous foreboding of the absurdity of life.

Here was a Christian who looked things straight in the eye, who had acknowledge the new world that has grown up around us, and who was willing to take a starting-point in these realities for a serious evaluation. Like the old parish shepherd he also was, death was perhaps not taboo nor at all remote to him.

The Catholics, as opposed to our Protestant pastors, have kept their old custom of following their flock directly into death. So Rieber-Mohn lived in both the old *and* the new worlds.

Chapter Three

Just after Easter – Wednesday the sixth of April, at
quarter past nine – I was back at Ullevål Hospital
again, at the Radiotherapy Department. I had been
sent a small pink card for Easter, stating time and
place, and which also said I was to go to the
'Simulator'. That was for preparatory markings
before the actual radium treatment.

After I had sat waiting for a while out in the
corridor, I was fetched by a young special nurse and
taken to a relatively large room containing a whole
row of technical-medical installations. The nurse
turned out to be Swedish. He must have been in his
early twenties, neat and well-trained, a picture of well-
built youth. Unassuming, and at the same time open
and friendly.

I was nervous, unusually nervous actually,
shutting myself behind a rather resigned and certainly
not a very merry mask. But the young Swede made me
relax.

I noticed this with some surprise. During my time at Ullevål Hospital, I came across several of these young men, and I was struck by the quite natural masculine gentleness they possessed. Men are also capable of care, and of discreet, unassuming consideration.

On the whole, I have been much struck by the way Norway has changed since I was a child, how the conventional and stereotyped division of the sexes is disappearing in many places, most striking of all perhaps in this hospital environment. This young Swede was like a mother hen, just like the authoritative sisters; explaining and helping me to recover.

I was installed on a kind of wheeled bed, and he started adjusting his apparatus according to a schedule he had presumably fetched from my file. I was given a thorough explanation of the procedure that entailed my having to be prepared to lie without moving for quite long periods of time, so that they could adjust the apparatus finely on exactly the areas where the radiation was to be directed. That was three places: two on the right side of my upper torso and one on the right side of my back.

After a while, a woman came into the room, said good-morning to me – taking my immobile right hand in a kind of greeting, introducing herself and asking me not to move. She was the doctor.

I suppose I lay without moving for something like three quarters of an hour all told. Without the nurse's and the doctor's calming and, at the same time, professional conduct, I don't think I would have managed it.

It is truly difficult to lie without moving at all, to order. I knew that I had all of twenty-five sessions ahead of me, for about five weeks, every single weekday, during which I was to lie immobile under this amazing apparatus, if only for a few minutes at a time. So I tried to find some kind of system within myself, something I could attach myself to in a relaxed way.

It meant lying under the simulator and letting yourself sink into total passivity, and simultaneously keeping your nerves in check with an intense preoccupation with what was going on all around.

And that was certainly not a little. The apparatus buzzed. Lights winked and I think little bells also rang. I was wheeled into the various positions relative to the apparatus. Bright red lines were painted on me, the young Swede working with a kindly hand, and afterwards I felt like an Indian woman covered in war-paint.

I was also photographed with an apparently perfectly ordinary camera, and finally I was tattooed. Tiny little black tattooed spots marked out strategic corners of this war-paint on my body. All this was to ensure that the schedule the radiation was to follow would be visible in the long five weeks it was to last.

This thing they called the 'Simulator' turned out to be an apparatus which, to me anyhow, looked approximately like the real radiation apparatus I was to be treated with. As usual, this calmed me.

I have noticed generally that what is most frightening in illness is anything quite new. If it is something recognizable, anxiety soon disperses. You get used to everything. Absolutely everything, I expect.

So the day after my confrontation with the simulator, when I went into a room farther down the corridor, where the proper radium treatment was to

76

take place, I at once saw that it was familiar from the day before, so it did not frighten me.

Blessed simplicity, you might say. I felt I 'recognized this'. In reality, I understood nothing of this complicated machinery, and at that particular time, I tried to avoid even asking questions. Much later, I tried to read myself into some kind of understanding from my famous cancer book, and although I recognized some of it, I have to admit I have an intellectual hostility to going into the scientific details of 'high-voltage apparatus', 'isode graphs' and 'radiation-bundles', just to name some of the words I came across in my reading.

I should have thought my intellect would be capable of, if not *understanding* all this, at least acquiring a reasonable *grasp* of what it was all about. But I still recoil with considerable aversion . . .

During my first radiotherapy session, which lasted for five or six minutes, in two doses, I contented myself with registering the huge apparatus. It was a large, heavy kind of crane under which I was placed on a mobile bed. Two special nurses adjusted my position in relation to a large tube from this crane, in which they had placed something that looked like glass plates with lead or other forms of metal on them. With the help of electronic instruments, the distance between my body and this point on the crane was adjusted millimetre by millimetre. When the two nurses were ready with the positioning, which they carried out with very swift routine movements, they indicated to me that they were now going to leave the room. I must not move for two or three minutes: radiation was about to begin.

They also told me there was contact between me

and the room outside, via television and microphones, so if I wanted anything, all I had to do was to say so. They wanted to hear and see me, and be able to talk to me. Then they disappeared out of the room.

A few seconds went by, during which I lay immobile. Then a quiet humming started in the huge apparatus, and apart from that, I noticed nothing. Absolutely nothing. No smell, nothing visible happening, just a slight hum.

I managed to lie still relatively easily for those two to three minutes. But I noticed that I tensed horribly, out of fear of moving, and it was a relief when the door opened and the two nurses came back in again.

Then the positioning began all over again, but now in a different position, and there was a change of glass plates and metal pieces. Then another session of two to three minutes of total immobility.

This became the routine, for twenty-five sessions, over a period of five weeks. Every fifth session, I had an extra dose, on my back.

I cannot say this really frightened me. It was mostly quite unreal. Unfathomable. I knew my body was being 'pumped full' of something that was extremely deadly, and that you felt nothing, smelt nothing, saw nothing. All this was to cure me.

I also soon found out that it would be difficult to endure these remarkable and totally meaningless circumstances, I mean remarkable and meaningless purely psychically speaking, every single day for weeks, if I didn't find some way of facing up to them. My interest in what was actually happening, in the apparatus and the nurses too – intellectual curiosity over it – disappeared, because I had to concentrate on finding a way of lying still without my reactions ending in some form of panic, something I did not think was entirely inconceivable.

This was when something happened to me which was quite elementary but also had a touch of irony about it. As I mentioned before, I had my daily dose of twice three minutes of immobility underneath the great apparatus. Relax was the keyword. But how?

Thinking about something else is an old trick. I had one method I had used for years, which I always tried if I had rare spells of insomnia. Many years ago, a friend of mine advised me to 'count the sheep of Iceland'. This entailed imagining Iceland, then seeing in front of your eyes a huge flock of sheep and starting to count the individual sheep in this flock.

This could lead to many miraculous futilities, in which one's thoughts and mind wandered over an imaginary landscape in Iceland in search of imaginary sheep. Thus one fell asleep from sheer monotonous peacefulness, but also perhaps because topical thoughts or problems that are apt to grow into monsters when insomnia afflicts you, become pushed to one side by imaginary sheep.

But this was not much use here. This was when the book on Buddhism I happened to have found in a city bookshop came into the picture.

I had noticed a number of descriptions of various Buddhist methods of what I would call 'spiritual gymnastics'. All of them put great emphasis on *breathing*. I had also noticed that both the physiotherapist I had at Ullevål and the one I went to several times a week in my own street, also talked about 'breathing well' or 'breathing out', or 'don't forget your breathing'. This had let me to discover that in many difficult situations, I actually stopped breathing.

As both distant Buddhists and Norwegian physiotherapists are so concerned with breathing, then there must be something in it, I thought, as I kept trying to relax underneath the radiation apparatus.

Buddhists think that the 'vital centre' in a human being is not the brain, as we usually presume, but in an area somewhere between the navel and the pelvis. In the abdomen. One of their methods entails 'making contact' with this vital centre.

The famous lotus position so often found in Asian art, both in paintings and sculpture, is for this purpose. During the thirty years or so I lived in France, I must have seen hundreds of Indian, Japanese or south-east Asian portrayals of Buddha, some of them among the wonders of world art. Like most people, I was naturally struck by the effect of complete composure these sculptures and paintings have.

Composure, yes. That was just what I felt I had to find in my daily struggle with immobility beneath this huge machine. The labyrinths of the mind are indeed unfathomable. I had read one of Buddha's own expressions in the book on Buddhism that stuck in my mind, I think out of pure intellectual interest.

It was something like this – 'Buddha is yourself.' This interested me, as I explained earlier, because of what I think about Christianity and its pretensions to order and the strong contrast presented by Buddhism.

Something like – do not seek for answers outside yourself; do not seek happiness in some Utopian paradise beyond this earth; seek inside yourself. I was struck by the similarity with Socrates, who lived at about the same period of time, but in another part of the world, and his (or Plato's) 'perceive yourself'. But these were more intellectual interests.

However, I suddenly said to myself that perhaps this was a way to calm myself down when I was beneath that machine. So I took the book on Buddhism and sat down on the floor of my own sitting-room at home and tried out the famous lotus position.

It turned out not to be an easy position to sit in, and my stiff infirmity caused me to burst out laughing. Your back should be quite straight. That was all right up to a point. Then your legs should be crossed, your knees never higher than your hips.

I never got my knees right. The hand position with the back of your left hand placed in the palm of your right hand, thumbs touching – that was relatively easy.

Then there were your eyes. They should not be closed, but 'veiled'. Your gaze should be turned down, fixed just beyond the tip of your nose. That went well, too. Then you take a deep breath, right down from your stomach.

I was not altogether successful at these exercises, but they interested me because I noticed they banished the constantly uneasy thoughts from my mind. So I amused myself with this, and at that time I did indeed need something to amuse me.

Well, I was no Buddha, even if the blessed Buddha had said that 'Buddha is yourself'. But what was the purpose of these exercises, from a Buddhist point of view?

The main idea is that our 'ego', our dominating consciousness of ourselves – which becomes almost obsessive during illness – has to learn to 'abandon itself', as it is called, to enable you to 'strike root in life itself'. That is, strike root in the larger context, in nature and the universe, of which the Buddhists think we are an integral part. The purpose of the exercises is to learn to 'let things go'. You have to 'give way', to 'accept' and 'trust', rather than 'cling to', 'hold on to' and 'control'.

I must admit that although such thoughts interested me in many ways, I did not get very far. I was, and still am, perfectly aware of the fact that the Buddhist system requires years of practice, and includes many other phenomena apart from the lotus position. I probably take a rather similar neutral attitude to this view of life as I do to other religions. But I was clutching at straws, for myself.

What calmed me most was this fixing a veiled look on the end of my nose and breathing in, deeply, evenly and rhythmically. When black thoughts came sweeping over me, on sleepless nights after nightmares, at home or elsewhere, I took up this method and it turned out to be very effective. It calmed me.

After a few days of radiotherapy sessions, from which I had emerged exhausted from tensing my muscles, I tried the method out there, too. And it worked. It was quite fantastic.

Then it became routine. I went into the radiotherapy room, smiled at the two nurses waiting for me, took off my hospital jacket, got up on to the bed, settled in the position the nurses requested, then half-closed my eyes and fixed my gaze just beyond the tip of my nose.

From then on I lay immobile, breathing deeply and rhythmically. And my whole body relaxed. My head was empty of thoughts. My mind was free of fear. When the two sessions of three minutes' radiation were over, I got up, said goodbye to the two nurses, put on the hospital jacket again, went out to the little booth in the corridor and dressed.

Thus the days went by. After finding this breathing-trick of mine, I managed to keep myself reasonably well under control. I had learnt something from this. All you have to do is to give in. So to some extent, I managed to keep the whole gigantic hospital system slightly at a distance.

Even the semi-dark radiotherapy room gradually became almost familiar and dear to me. I could lie with my eyes half-closed, watching the two nurses positioning me and the instruments, finding that I was observing something as distant as a nurse's hand holding a small apparatus and pressing a little button to move the bed I was lying on. Or I might observe with complete calm the new hair-do of one of the nurses.

I hardly ever spoke to them, and neither did they say much, except for good-morning and thank you when I left. The nurses were usually always the same ones, except once or twice when they had the day off.

I know their faces. I know what their hands look like. I have observed them at close quarters for so long that if I were to meet one of them in the street one day, I think I would probably imagine she was a close friend of mine . . . But in truth, I have hardly ever spoken to them. I was probably just one of many to them, many people in a routine they carried out all day long, about every ten minutes.

They were particularly friendly, as was everyone I came into contact with. That is not the point. Friendly, caring and considerate. But both they and I were parts of a huge machinery. We were cogs in a complicated and almost unfathomable machine that kept grinding on and on, day and night.

We were close to each other, and at the same time so distant, as if we were objects, not people. So it was almost a shock when occasionally one of us, they or I, broke the routine and said something.

I remember one such occasion with great delight. It was the ordinary routine – I went in, lay down, was given radiotherapy and got down off the bed. Then as she helped me off the bed, I heard the gentlest of the two nurses say: 'Well, that was today's little dash . . . '

I laughed. And she laughed. Then we were suddenly two people meeting, open and merry, quite unconnected with the machinery. I shall probably remember 'today's little dash' as long as I live, for one is so vulnerable and wretched in the world of hospitals that things etch themselves on your mind, perhaps most of all 'happy moments' which tell you that you are still a human being.

The world of hospital. By definition it is not a happy world for patients. Naturally, those who earn their livings in the profession and so also live in that world together with us patients, like it and can be very happy in it. It also helps a little that there are so many contented people bustling about the corridors all the time.

I remember sitting out in the corridor one day in the surgical department, together with a row of other, much more seriously ill men and women. There was a sudden burst of laughter and men's voices at the end of the corridor. A crowd of young men in white doctor's coats came towards us, talking animatedly. With smiles and laughter and energetic strides, the whole crowd swept past us, literally flowing with youthful contentment.

But this is a world a patient only catches a glimpse of now and again. You mostly encounter long rows of patients, as I did in the radiology department.

There were two treatment rooms there, the second clearly a replica of the one I went to daily. My appointment was at nine o'clock every weekday, and as I walked along the passage, I always saw rows of people waiting. There were often bed-patients too, who had been wheeled down from other departments, or possibly out-patients wheeled in from an ambulance that had brought them from home.

Some were like myself, relatively mobile. Others were obviously much more seriously ill. I had the feeling as I had had in the surgical unit that 'my case' was of a less critical nature.

I don't really think that helped much. As the treatment progressed, my awareness of the fact that I had a disease with many and unpredictable chances of recurrence increased. The sight of critically ill people sends ominous feelings through you, although compassion for others also helps you to be able to see yourself more realistically and to get things into proper proportion.

I had my fixed routine. Arriving at Ullevål at almost exactly nine o'clock every morning, I swung in through the swing-door of what is called the Middle Block, turned left and walked down the long corridor to the Radiotherapy Department, which was on the left of the passage.

It went like clockwork. I went into the passage

outside the radiotherapy room. Four or five people might be sitting there waiting. I went straight to one of the series of booths in the corridor to undress – a little room containing a chair, a mirror, a hook, just adequate for an adult to stand up in and undress, with a curtain you could draw across.

I took a blue and white striped hospital jacket down from a large shelf, stripped to the waist, put the jacket on and went out into the corridor to wait. That usually only took a few seconds, for I was becoming almost manic in my daily routine.

After radiation, I went back to the booth, dressed, threw the blue and white jacket into a large laundry basket, went over to a table where there was a jug of blackcurrant juice, drank a cup of it, then left, down the corridor, turn right, down the long passage and out of the hospital again.

Now and again this manic routine might be broken. There were days, for instance, when for one reason or another there were queues of bed-patients, usually a sad sight. These were people who could not stand and had to be wheeled to radiotherapy. On those days, the nurses' appointments with us ordinary walking patients were thrown into confusion and then I had to sit in the corridor and wait.

I remember very well one of those days, because I witnessed one of those episodes that make such a strong impression in this world of the sick. Seeing people so exhausted that you can hardly grasp that they are alive is almost solemn. Human misery, with death and obliteration, is overwhelming.

That day there was a bed standing by the door to the radiotherapy room, a young nurse at the foot of it, wheeling it carefully aside. A person lay in the bed, a man, an old man, an infinitely aged man, I would say.

But how old was he really? Cancer ages people dramatically when it is as critical as this. So what did I know about this man's age?

I felt the man was only connected with life by a few fragile little threads. He was lying with his eyes half-closed, an intravenous drip attached to several parts of his body, and he was terribly thin and pale. He groaned now and again, or breathed an exhausted sigh.

The nurse constantly attended him, asking him how he was. He never answered, perhaps never even heard.

A young doctor came and leant over the man and said something to him, then started talking quietly and gently to him, something about how he was. There was no reply.

The doctor looked up and stood there without moving for a few seconds, glancing up and down the corridor. Then he bent down over the man again and said: 'You needn't go in. We'll stop the treatment for today.'

There was apparently no reaction from the man. But the doctor leant over him and put his ear to his face. He may have heard the man say something, for he nodded and said: 'Yes, yes.' Then there was movement everywhere, the bed was wheeled away and sisters and nurses came out of the radiotherapy room to arrange things with the waiting patients.

I sat there watching the man being wheeled away, so absorbed in this drama that had been played out among us that I never heard when the sister called me and said: 'It's your turn'. I shook off those strong impressions, took a deep breath and went in for my daily routine, into the radiotherapy room, off with my jacket, down on the bed, then fixing my veiled gaze just beyond my nose and breathing deeply . . .

My solution to these daily radiotherapy sessions was to abandon myself to the routine. When the day's 'dash' was over, I hesitantly and cautiously tried to find my way back to a zest for life I felt I had largely lost. But the routine was a kind of daily prison existence. Every single day, I tried to break out of it the moment I strode firmly out of Middle Block at Ullevål. I then usually headed for the long avenue that runs down to Geitemyr Road.

But on some days I made my way rather hesitantly inside the gates of Ullevål Hospital, taking in the nearest buildings at first. I discovered a whole town inside its walls, a post office, a bank, a supermarket, and I also made use of the available services on some days.

The huge old trees of Ullevål were still fine, but they seemed overwhelmed by this world of machines and cars. The remains of the old hospital that was built at the beginning of the century were touching to see, but looked like doll's houses, the huge new buildings dominating them. I found these gigantic buildings of steel and glass almost frightening, but I constantly returned to them, standing there gazing at them, wondering what 'really' went on inside them, behind those sterile glassy facades.

One day I discovered something quite close to one of those glass towers – a downhill entrance for cars, grey all over, in so-called 'natural concrete', the ideological architectural fashion in Norway for most of the post-war period.

When I looked down this tunnel, I saw a series of aluminium racks and white glass globes. Clearly an entrance to something. Or was it the way out *from* something? For it was one-way traffic there, and instead of the usual red and white traffic sign, this one was *black and white.* It made a remarkable impression. I found a tiny notice which said: *To the Chapel.*

I stopped in my tracks and stared at it for a long time, then went the other way, thinking I would look at all that another time. Not today, another time.

Most days, however, I headed for the lovely old avenue that emerges by Nordre Gravlund, where Geitmyr Road starts. For I walked from Ullevål every day, taking about an hour to cover the distance to my own street in Vika.

I had been told that I must be sure to 'live a healthy life' while having radiotherapy, one of those rather vague generalizations that are not easy to understand. But I thought a daily walk in the fresh air must be healthy, and I like walking, the only kind of exercise I have taken over the last twenty years. I have been walking in the Norwegian and French mountains for years, and I am also a city walker. I have walked miles through the streets of Paris over the years, and now, in the spring of 1983, I was walking the streets of Oslo.

These daily walks from Ullevål were an attempt to free myself from the hospital world, which was increasingly oppressing me. Spring was late that year and it was cold and wet for a long time. But all through April and half of May, whether wet or sunny, whether cold or with a touch of spring in the air, I took my daily walk into the city. Everywhere, I heard people complaining about the bad spring, but to me it was a lovely time.

One's birthplace always remains within one in a very special way. Oslo is like that for me. The light in the streets at this time of year brings back strong memories in me.

I remembered my first bicycle, as a young girl. I remembered playing my first game of hopscotch after the snow had gone, and also tossing pennies, using five *øre* coins against a wall in Skov Road, where the asphalt had gone and the earth was showing through. I remembered how we stopped in a back yard on our way home from school and got out our scrap-books and compared glossy scraps. And I remembered we collected cigarette cards – caricatures by Kloumann and race-horses were my speciality . . .

On these daily walks through the streets, I also realized that as a child, I obviously never noticed whether or not spring had come. I lived for the present and took the weather and seasons as something constantly immediate, not as a unity or a development. Like a daily drop one took for something or other, spring or autumn, cold or hot.

It's not like that any longer, I thought. Now I see time in great chunks. 'Spring will soon be here', I say, for instance, and I try to follow the progress of the seasons in trees and gardens, in the light and the rain.

Neither is it a bad thing to be adult! The wealth of experience and memories an adult can draw on is copious, and as these memories and experiences started appearing in my thoughts on my daily walks, I began a systematic voyage of discovery in a part of

Oslo I had known really quite well as a child, but also knew very little about.

One of my great discoveries was Uranienborg Terrace, which lies beyond Uranienborg Church. 'Beyond' here means that the boundary of my childhood world was Uranienborg Church. I never went any further. This is connected with the strong territorial world of childhood, and now, as an adult, I discovered an amazingly delightful part of Oslo, full of old wooden houses and lovely gardens. The fact that all this had been there near the streets I used daily as a child was hard to believe; so my childhood kingdom had been that small.

But that small childhood world had gone on being very large inside me. I began to walk systematically through it. I visited Uranienborg Church – but of course could not go inside, owing to the dismal habit Protestants have of locking churches when no service is being held. In my mind, this church is larger than Notre Dame in Paris, so perhaps it was just as well that I couldn't get in. This was where we children at Uranienborg School went every year to a service on the last day of term before Christmas, and it was in this church that I sang 'The bells do ring, yes, ring for day in the half-light' for the very first time. I remember it as a magnificent occasion.

I also went inside my old Uranienborg School, down the corridors, across the school playground, looking into the caretaker's quarters. I felt like a giant in the land of Lilliputians. Everything was so small, and the school track down to Skov Road, on the corner of Frogner Road, was so short. Not to mention how small the back yard in Behren Street was, which I remembered as a huge open space.

* * *

I dreamt my way away from the hospital and illness. Perhaps it was the knowledge that spring was just round the corner that gave me such pleasure on these daily rounds. I am not sure if it would have been the same being ill in the autumn, when one would know winter lay ahead with its long cold darkness.

This waiting for spring and summer produced such a zest for life that it was easy to imagine myself quite healthy. I got through those weeks in April and May by working up some of my old *joie de vivre*, from one moment to the next. I felt that nature, with her driving, inflexible course, was seizing me and sending me on downstream, just as rivers do with everything that gets in the way in spring.

Now and again I went to art exhibitions, one of which I shall not forget in a hurry. Or rather, a picture in one of these exhibitions. It was at the Kunsternes Hus gallery. The exhibition was of a selection from the great Youth Biennial that had been held in Paris. The picture was by a young Frenchwoman, one of those modern works that can be called neither a painting nor a photograph, but is a kind of collage. But it was not the form that was important. It was the content that transfixed me.

The picture was about fifteen feet long, a rather blurred photo-montage in black and white, in *ice-cold* black and white, portraying an unconscious woman on an operating table, her head turned to the right, surrounded by all kinds of apparatus, bound by a series of leads to her body.

I was startled. It was as if this French artist had taken her photo-montage straight out of my own

92

nightmares. So this was so common that a totally strange woman in Paris could conjure it up again before my own eyes . . .

I went round the exhibition several times, but kept coming back to this picture. It both attracted and repelled me at the same time. It is true that such pictures are a kind of therapy. I know exactly what this woman artist had worked with. I have never seen anything else by her. I don't know who she is. But one thing I do know – I would never want to have such a picture in my home. It *is* therapy. Can one live with therapy in one's own home? Isn't that like bringing the hospital world back home?

There is a great deal in modern art that borders on therapy, so perhaps the world appears sick to many artists. I went back to that picture several times, and I felt the 'benefit' of it to me, of having nightmare images made concrete, brought out into the light and consciousness. This doesn't make them any less nightmarish, but they at least acquire realistic proportions; though still not anything I would want on the sitting-room wall at home in Vika.

Why not? Something was missing from the picture, as in so much of today's art.

I hesitate to use the word. It is a word that is despised, misused and worn out with speculation and philistinism. But I will do so all the same – beauty. It is beauty that is missing in many of these therapeutic pictures.

Rembrant's 'The Anatomy Lesson' suddenly appears in my mind – the male corpse in the middle of the picture and the students and teachers around it. A dramatic and really rather horrible subject. But it is not horrible. Why not? I think it is simply because there is beauty in it.

This is not aesthetics, not banal beauty for enjoyment. It is a dimension beyond the physical. So instead of being therapy for crippled human beings, it is charisma. Suffering and death and what is frightening about a person cutting into a dead person are transformed into something else. The picture becomes 'an answer', beyond reality and logic, an answer to the question one asks about what is frightening one.

This is the form of beauty I so often find lacking in the art I see today. On the other hand, I do find this beauty in nature, and not just in sunlight. I find it in animals, in their 'innocent' animal conduct. That is what I have always sought in art, poetry and music, and during this spring of 1983, I felt more than ever in need of just that.

More than faith, more than the assurance that I would get better, more than the care and concern of friends and relatives, it was this charisma in beauty that was my greatest need. I needed it to counter the daily walk into the hospital world, with all its misery and machines and incomprehensible means of progress.

It seemed to me that it was the human being in me, the woman in me – independent of this miserable body of mine – that was struggling to survive. I refused to be a PATIENT, a number, a body that had taken over.

But that miserable body was there, making its considerable demands. I had very little surplus vitality. Not that radiotherapy brought with it any of the things the doctors had said *might* happen. I did not feel particuarly nauseated. I did not have any blisters, nor headaches worth mentioning. But I became easily depressed and suffered from a vague mental exhaustion.

The only thing I was really able to manage was the trip to Ul/evål every day and the walk back home to Vika afterwards, with some diversions into new and old Oslo, or a few exhibitions. The thought of doing any work, by which I mean writing articles for the papers or completing my latest book, evoked sheer nausea, and the world of politics, at home and abroad, that had occupied me all my life filled me with a kind of dreadful loathing . . .

Apart from my daily trips to the hospital, I also went three times a week to the physiotherapist in my own locality. That soon became a faint light in the tunnel of physical misery I was in. The persistent stiffness in my right side dominated my whole life. Walking, standing and lying – everything was determined by this stiff deadness in my body, as well as a certain fear of moving naturally. I had a manic, probably exaggerated fear of what might happen to the wound.

At the physiotherapist's this was soon brought under control. Regular treatment to my arm and the areas round it, together with her and my own increasingly bolder traction of the arm and shoulder had surprisingly swift results. This was basically the first encouraging sign since the operation.

My physiotherapist was a mature, professional, and at the same time, unassuming person. Caring was perhaps the right word. For in contrast to the Ulleval nurses, she was far from silent. She talked on and on. So caring was probably the word.

Caring of the *person* I was, more than the body I also was. For she was not afraid to pull and stretch at my arm, whereas I shrank in terror at the first unexpected movement. I discovered with great relief that it went well, that I could also stretch and move my arm, gradually more and more assuredly.

Things went ahead from day to day with seven-league strides. I was as proud as Punch when I could lift my right arm above my nose, not to mention when I managed to get it up above my head.

So the sessions with the physiotherapist came to mean much more to me than physical training back to normal. It was a place where things were obviously *progressing*, where I could actually take things into my own hands and haul myself up out of the world of the sick. I enjoyed the sessions, in contrast to my slavish trip to Ullevål to which I had adapted and become resigned.

The sessions were like small white stones in my black landscape, small symbols of life returning. My physiotherapist was with me all the way, encouraging me, boasting about me, probably much more than was really warranted.

I have never been particularly athletic, so my physical achievements have never been very impressive. When I looked at her and noticed how trim and healthy and physically well-adjusted she was, there were occasions when I looked at myself with a certain tristesse. But never for one moment did I ever have the feeling that I shocked her with my wretched carved-up body.

I suppose they get used to physical wretchedness, these physiotherapists, and effortlessly manage to look at us soberly, without involvement. Whatever it is, it was important to me that I saw no kind of terror in the eyes of the physiotherapist, nor any resigned pessimism. Neither did this ever happen to me, despite the fact that my perceptions were sharpened by suspicion. My respect for the physiotherapist's profession greatly increased over this period of time.

So this was the place where I found a way out of my misery. 'The place' was in fact an old Kristiania apartment in Vika, and compared with Ulleval and all its technical and material wonders, it was touchingly antiquated, which goes to show that equipment is perhaps not always of greatest importance, anyway, not for patients. People are more important, and the circumstances, of course.

My circumstances pointed in the direction of possible improvement, which made the cramped quarters less important. Maybe everything in the radiotherapy and other departments at Ulleval also pointed to a cure for me, but I was not in a position to judge. That was all abstract. A young doctor had indeed said to me once, when I had a 'telephone appointment' with him, that 'when the radiotherapy was over I could regard myself as cured'.

That was easy to say. How could I know that? I had never yet even felt ill or that I had cancer, so how would I one day be able to feel I was well and no longer had it?

Here, on the other hand, in this cramped little room, lying on a bed behind a curtain in the physiotherapy institute, I literally felt that I *would* get better. Cured was another matter. But I felt my muscles being stretched and made to function again. I felt my whole right side, which had been ripped up and sliced up and down and across through nerves, sinews and arteries, would be able to function again.

I got the sessions with the physiotherapist through my health insurance, via the surgeon who had operated on me. After a while, I had used up my ration, a fact the physiotherapist brought to my attention and asked me whether I could manage on my own from then on.

I seemed to be panic-stricken by the thought. A feverish energy came over me, as if it were a matter of life and death. She looked rather frightened, but told me that if I felt I needed to go on, that would be no problem. All I had to do was to ask the doctor for further appointments. I was determined to go on and pay for myself if necessary.

This feverish reaction surprised even myself. It revealed my need for 'everything to go well.' Not since I was a child, or a youngster, have I felt such a burning desire as this need to continue with the physiotherapist.

Illness is truly a remarkable affair. One becomes like a helpless child again, or a vulnerable young girl. I think I probably scared the physiotherapist with my violent reaction. Purely objectively, there were probably no real grounds for my continuing with her. But the next time I went to Ulleval, I went to the surgical clinic to get a doctor's note. I really did feel it was a matter of life and death.

I have to smile when I think back on it. It is no easy matter simply getting through to a busy doctor in a department where there is a queue of people waiting. But the sister took one look at me and said without hesitating – 'I'll fix it for you.'

I was overwhelmed with gratitude, and when the doctor's own sister came out ten minutes later with the note, tears gushed uncontrollably down my cheeks.

The sister looked at me and smiled, with perhaps some slight confusion, or perhaps she was quite used to crazy patients like me. Anyhow, I got my new note and went regularly to the physiotherapist's marvellously 'healing' and optimistic sessions for a few more weeks.

Saturdays and Sundays were free days from radio-therapy at Ullevål. Then I was looked after by the person closest to me and we drove together up the Sørkedalen valley to Skansebakken, where we parked the car. Then we walked on.

I don't think there is anywhere else in the world I feel closer to than the tracks and paths there, the beginnings of Krokskogen woods. It all seems to be linked in my mind with Asbjørnsen's wanderings and fairy tales, as well as my own excursions both in summer and winter as a child, as a younger woman, and all through my life. If there is, then it's the great deciduous woods north of Paris. Endless birchwoods, with trunks and crowns like cathedrals, where you can walk for hours without meeting a soul, and where the magical light through the leaves plays on your imagination. But that kingdom of light and fertile greenery, that ethereal miracle is a much more recent experience than the much darker and sterner Krokskogen of my childhood.

Along the tracks and paths in from Skanse-bakken, it was like coming home again that spring of 1983.

I know this countryside like the back of my hand, so that it almost hurts at the moment of recognition. For what did the illness I had just been through actually mean to me? It meant that the whole of my life came rushing in on me again, in clear persistent images. Not always with delight, either. What had happened to that inflexible faith I had once had? What had really happened to me? Had all that toil and strife been really worth while?

A kind of painful bitterness can also well up inside you . . . how little you have 'got out of' or 'made of' all the endless things that once long ago lay ahead, when you first walked these paths and smelt the thawing snow and rotting leaves, or stopped for the first time in front of those rosy stony slopes that are the brilliant jewels of the outskirts of Oslo. And you remember the naïve infinite faith from a youth that was hard enough in many ways, but which was totally unaware of the slow disintegration of everything, even your actual zest for life.

One of the popular tunes at the time came to me one day as we were strolling along the damp paths across from Skansebakken – 'I never promised you a rose garden . . . ' The song means something quite different, but that line came to mean something quite special to me.

No one had ever promised me, or anyone else, a rose garden. I repeated it over and over again to myself. Who do you really think you are? But human arrogance, the apparently firm belief that we have been 'promised something' is stronger than reason and causes this vague painful bitterness.

What our life *is*, what is concrete and realistically near, is never enough. There is always something else, something inexpressible perhaps, that we feel we can demand. And then when one day we are suddenly faced with the black wall that the thought of death is to most of us, we cry over 'our wasted life'.

It was always only during the first half-hour or so along the paths that such wildly contradictory thoughts ran round my head.

Walking, walking oneself into another world. Walking out of yourself.

This is no doubt something purely physiological. A friend of mine who knows all about these crude physical matters has tried to explain for years what happens when the blood circulation starts up in the body, and the different chemical processes that begin functioning. I have probably never had the patience to understand any of it.

But I do know something significant happens when you go out walking, and so go out of yourself, and literally into the countryside. For me, the explanation for this is quite unscientific and is that you come closer to the beauty to be found in the simultaneously brutal and miraculously harmonious countryside, which is also utterly uninterested in your own small self.

That was what it was like.

The blue ridges along from Sørkedalen valley, the last remaining red-painted farms in the distance, the bare white birch trees on the horizon, topped with the purplish veil of the silhouettes of their leafless crowns, and the gloomy, heavy black spruces, the gloomiest trees in the world!

Of all the coniferous trees, I think I really prefer pines. I prefer their pine haze, their much more optimistic elegance . . . But no. The solemn spruces are my world, the world with which and from which I was born.

That spring of 1983, along the very paths where I was walking, the spruces had their flowering year. The great pink 'flowers', or whatever this fertility feast of the spruce can be called, glowed at us from every spruce top, the pollen covering the paths and tracks with its golden blanket.

One day, I was standing on a hill above Slora, looking across the hills to the west. The weather was fresh and changeable, wild dark clouds racing across the sky and gusts of wind swirling over the ridges.

Then a kind of transparent curtain rose up across the landscape, as far as the eye could see towards the distant horizon. A shower, I thought. A shower racing across the hills. But no. It was a dust-cloud of spruce pollen moving across the dark forest like a silken veil, like an airborne dance. It lasted a few seconds, then the dark forests lay there again, heavy and silent.

Yes. The fresh air, 'the healthy life', as the hospital would call it, or the beauty of the countryside so close to my heart, which in my unscientific way I preferred to call it, was of a healing kind.

I don't say 'curing'. Fundamentally I had fewer and fewer illusions over whether I would ever have any guarantee that one day, any day, I would not die of cancer. It was the black wall that never went away.

But gradually, I slowly began to adapt, in spite of it, perhaps because of it, to the *moment* always being there – the blessed present. On these country walks even the gloomy spruces could produce a miracle for me that was worth a small eternity.

The scientific and physical world of hospital would no doubt explain that I had lactic acid in my blood and so had produced energy for myself . . . I felt I had caught hold of a scrap of something that could give me back my zest for life, and that was enough for me.

I always came back to my apartment in Vika after these walks with a feeling of being almost 'normal' again.

* * *

My slave routine at Ullevål soon brought me down to earth again. There were so many *impressions*.

One day, for instance, there was an infant. An infant with cancer! I saw the man carrying the tiny creature in his arms, and the woman behind him, on their way into the treatment room. At such moments, death wrapped itself round me like an icy bag that I had no possible chance of getting out of, threatening to suffocate me.

Fantasies! Nightmare thoughts! With words like that I shook off these impressions, but I never got away from the picture of that little baby.

My own various examinations were also more prosaic. They checked my blood and were constantly examining it. But there were other tests, too, and one day I was given a small pink card by the sister in the radiotherapy department.

On it was – 'Isotope, 14/4, 9.30 a.m. Bring sandwiches. The examination takes a long time.' And on the back, it said: 'Mammography, Thursday, 12/4. 8.45 a.m.'

Good heavens! This was an earthquake in my brittle little routine world. What was up now? I went off to this new item feeling the sheep-instinct of the early days of my illness had got hold of me again.

'Mammography' turned out to be somewhere near the top of the building and I made my way there like a sleepwalker at exactly 8.45. A sturdy cheerful nurse received me, told me to strip to the waist and directed me towards another unfamiliar machine.

'Haven't you been here before?' the nurse said in surprise. No, I hadn't. 'They call it the meat-press,' she said, smiling warmly at me. That helped a little. The juicy humour found in professional worlds – its origins undoubtedly in the popular and disrespectful linguistic tradition of patients – really clears the air. Self-absorption and self-pity evaporate, and it feels like a good cold shower.

The 'meat-press' turned out to be simply a way of examining my remaining and hopefully healthy breast. The procedure was that I stood upright close to a large apparatus and placed my left breast inside a 'press', which was really an instrument for X-raying the breast. It was simple. Totally harmless. Not even unpleasant.

As soon as it was over the sheep in me had gone and I walked with firm brisk steps out of the department, down to my daily radiotherapy treatment, on to the bed, breathing deeply and listening to the humming of the machine.

'Isotope' turned out to be more elaborate and much more remarkable. This was to take place in a department parallel to the radiotherapy department, a passage I had glanced into so many times with a sense that something horrible probably happened *there*.

I was there at exactly half past nine on the day. I hadn't brought any sandwiches with me because I had asked the nurse and been told that the 'long time' the examination was to take involved having an injection of something (radioactive isotope!) which needed time to spread round my body, and that took a few hours. However, I could do what I liked during those hours, so I decided to go into town and come back again, rather than sit with sandwiches in the corridors of Ulleval. So I was given my injection and left.

A few hours later, I was back again. I was taken

into a room containing the usual bed and the inevitable huge incomprehensible machine. However, this time I did not have to undress. I lay down fully clothed and the huge machine was placed above my body.

What were they doing? A handsome young technician told me they were photographing my skeleton! 'Right through my clothes?' I asked. 'Yes,' he said, smiling in a slightly blasé way. And *that*'s what they did.

This was a 'gamma camera' a scanner, which was now localizing the injected radio-isotopes. This is called 'bone scanning'. They scanned the whole of my skeleton to check that this indeterminate disease was not 'lying in wait' somewhere else in my organism.

This was nothing to make a fuss about, either. I was used to lying beneath large machines every day, so it was pure routine. But there was something different – a sense of unreality . . . the way they 'see' through you . . . briefly, the incomprehensible hospital world.

One feels small in the hospital world, like a grain of sand, and for that reason I was often full of conflicts. I was both able to sink into the routine and literally *become* that grain of sand. Or submit to the sheep-like atmosphere.

Modern medicine's almost miraculous progress presupposed this enormous apparatus, and, of course, you want to get better, if necessary, against all odds. On top of that, none of this was the 'fault' of the doctors and nurses. Nor the 'fault' of these remarkable machines, either. But there were days when protest welled up in me, blind rage, really. But in the realities of modern Norway, I am not sure whether it could be done in any other way, taking into consideration the huge numbers of people the system has to deal with.

On cancer alone, what had I read in that official publication? Fourteen thousand new cases of cancer occur every year! I read the following sober medical estimates that of every fourth Norwegian, forty per cent can reckon on being cured. Forty-five per cent survive five years after treatment. Of these, eighty-six per cent will be alive twenty years later. (That is the only optimistic figure you can cling to.)

No, I don't think there is much to be gained by aiming your agitation and rage at the hospital world.

But there is a way in which this can find an outlet. As far as I was concerned, this manifested itself in often quite unreasonable bad temper I could not entirely control. Or else a great deal went *inwards*. You could call it melancholy, or self-pity of the vaguest possible kind; I let myself sink into the hospital routine, into my role as a grain of sand, or taking on that sheep-like nature.

Physical exhaustion probably played its part, but if the truth will out, the hospital and this passive resignation in myself also gave me a certain security. *That* troubled me in clearer moments, as it was quite new to me. I am not a particularly resigned person, and this capacity for passivity in myself was a terrible revelation.

That was when I was overcome with rage. I didn't really have either the physical or mental strength to break out of it altogether. But I told myself that the least I could do was to take my consciousness with me into this sinking world and try to *admit* what it is. In God's name live through yourself a little, and don't

106

just float along sleepwalker routines. I still had some of my old inquisitiveness, despite the fact that my zest for life had sunk to such a low level.

The most remarkable thing came to my rescue in all this agitation.

I have mentioned before that I have no particular faith in the Christian conviction that man is a kind of jewel in the universe, whom God in Heaven watches over in particular. On the contrary, I am probably one of those people who are struck by man's infinite loneliness faced with the incomprehensible and also probably unfathomable dimensions and multiplicity of the universe. Perhaps I am also one of those people who do not feel any particular agitation about that in itself. In that respect, I could perhaps be called a modern Stoic, an agnostic human being.

But this perception or 'belief' if you like, goes deeper than that in me. I have an intense feeling for the mystery of life. By that I mean that I regard feelings and perceptions as more 'real' than all the scientific 'discoveries' in the world.

Like most people of my day, I have tried as best I can to keep up with the progress of science both out in the universe as well as in the biological reality of our own planet, including mankind itself. I have been struck by the fact that all new gains – fascinating to me, anyhow, and filling me with an amazed admiration for this wonderful structure – always bring with them added problems.

It is like a magical system of boxes, in which each open box takes you on to an infinite series of new unopened boxes. I am not sure that it is possible for man to comprehend the universe. I think the mystery is beyond the biological capacity of mankind.

I don't think this view is one of fundamental resignation. I think a minute scrap of wisdom has brought me to that conclusion. I *accept* the mystery. I do not regard it as basically frightening, but as a wealth so great, a human life is insufficient to make the most of it, and my own messy life, should I now be granted life for twenty years after having cancer, would not be long enough to make me cynical.

The mystery is everywhere to me. That much despised word I used called beauty in art, poetry and music is, for instance, a mystery. But what about people? It's there in the astonishing things that arise between people: love, passion, friendship, concern, and in nature, where mystery is constantly present every single day. That is how it seems to me.

In the middle of the helpless passivity of my illness, it didn't take much to revive my interest in all this. There was, for instance, a small scene in my own backyard here in Vika that demanded neither too much of me, nor of my strength; the birds who came to my window.

All winter, I had put out a lump of fat mixed with seeds for them. I had hung the fat on a nail fairly high up on the window-frame outside, so that the crows and pigeons didn't take it in one gulp. This was for the little birds, and this winter the titmice came.

I had little energy left over for work, but nevertheless every day I spent a short time at my desk in my little study, where the tits' food was. Cautiously, I tried out some translation of poetry I had been working on for a long time.

These moments at my desk became spells with the birds. I observed them, and they were aware that I was there. Perhaps they were also observing me – I don't know how much birds see in the ordinary human sense.

So I might be sitting at my desk, totally absorbed in a phrase or expression, and I would hear thump-thump-thump from the nail outside the window. If I looked up, I could see either the tail of a tit, its head inside the lump, or I might see the top of its head sticking over the lump. Sometimes it would cease its feverish pecking at the lump, raise its head and look straight at me.

Did it see me? I don't know what birds see. In fact I soon found out I know very little about birds in general. But I saw its eyes, anyhow – deep, black, almost brilliant.

Animal eyes. Animal's eyes are a mystery to me.

I have encountered many animals in my life, cats as a child, but also cows, horses, sheep and hens. As a child, I imagined that those animal eyes spoke to me, just as we humans spoke with words. I am not so sure about that now, although I am fairly sure at least cats and dogs have the ability to express themselves with their eyes. I like to think so, anyhow.

But what about these tits on my windowsill? Were they expressing anything in relation to me, as I sat there at my desk? I thought so, but was never really sure.

The tiny blue-tits, which came very rarely, made a particular impression on me, for whether they were expressing anything to me or not, there was expression in their eyes.

What was it? It was the infinite loneliness of animals, the struggle for survival, the almost automatic anxiety, alertness, or caution when faced with anything that moved or made a sound. Now and again, as with the tiny blue-tits, I saw an infinite depth in their gaze when those two small eyes fastened on me over the edge of the lump of fat.

That was how I felt, as well as a kind of basic solidarity, an utterly illogical interdependence. If I were a grain of sand, I, a ridiculous human with all my arrogant pretensions, now almost sobbing before the great black wall that death was to me, then this was certainly nothing dramatic or new to the blue-tit. I followed its movements. What vitality! Against what odds? What quivering uncontrollable vigour.

As the weeks went by that spring, I also became convinced that this primaeval vitality in animals, which I suppose we tend to call instinctive, in contrast to our own vitality which is said to be 'divine', also had extremely individual and non-essential effects. I heard them twittering. I saw them swooping round marvellously in the spring sunshine. I became convinced that not *all* their twittering nor *all* those flying dances stemmed *only* from instinctive, automatic, biological needs.

I often went to the door of my study when I heard that thump-thump-thump from outside my window. The tits became for me a kind of first-aid in the struggle in my mind with my own sense of being a grain of sand. They brought something to life within me. What was it?

I realized one day with considerable surprise that they had quite simply transferred over to me that good old zest for life.

Wednesday, the eleventh of May was my last radio-therapy day. I was fairly worn out towards the end, both physically and spiritually, but it all finished in the same routine manner as it had begun.

In I went, out I went, with my usual brisk steps. I saw the surgeon who had operated on me and he fixed my appointment for a check-up for September. A fortnight later, I had to go to the radiologist for a check-up. 'How are things going?' she said.

I looked at her with a wry smile and said something about that I had no idea, but did she mean how was I? Yes, all was in order.

She looked at my papers. My blood was fine, and she added that should 'anything happen', well, then I must remember that 'we have ways of treating it'. She was a blessedly sane person who had helped me with her down-to-earth objectivity. I thanked her. Then I left.

It was now the twenty-seventh of June, sixteen weeks since the operation, almost four months. I had only one more thing to do at Ullevål, this time round, anyway. This was that tunnel down to the chapel, which I had decided to go and look at. I had set that up as a goal – I would pluck up my courage and go and look at it before I left Ullevål.

So I left the doctor's office, walked past the old Ullevål buildings towards the gigantic steel and glass block, and as if it were the most natural thing in the world, I walked down the concrete ramp.

I came to a glass door. It was locked, I think. I didn't actually try it, but I was sure it was locked. I stood there looking in at a wide concrete passage and reading the signs above.

On the left it said: 'Stop. No Entry'. On the right: 'Loading and Unloading'. There seemed to be an entrance on the other side as well, so I went round to try that one.

I met a thin bustling man on my way up. 'Are you looking for something?' he said. 'No,' I replied, and went on.

There was a similar ramp on the other side, up this time. Up only. But on this side the door was wide open, so I went inside. There was a notice: 'To the Chapel – 100 metres'. Slightly lower down it said: 'Pathology and Anatomy Laboratories'.

I walked across towards the chapel. On a door was: 'Microbiology Laboratory'. Inside a glass door lay a heap of large yellow sacks, and above them a notice: 'Not to be removed by Oslo City Cleansing Department.'

I had entered a medical factory – an icy, orderly underworld, I felt. I went on and came to a place with three notices. In the middle it said: 'Chapel', and on either side: 'Viewing Room 1' and 'Viewing Room 2'. I walked quietly over to the chapel door, opened it and went in – a tiny room, a catafalque in the middle and two or three chairs. That was all.

I slowly walked out again. I met no one. But just as I left the outer exit, I heard a car starting up behind me. A large glass door opened automatically and a car came out at top speed and drove off up the ramp. I caught a glimpse of a bareheaded young doctor in white clothes. He turned and looked at me as he drove past.

As usual, I walked back into the city that day, my last at Ulleval. I was feeling not a little proud of myself that I had gone down to the chapel.

One can clearly be filled with anxiety at the sight of a black and white traffic sign, when according to all the regulations it should be red and white. But I knew now that this famous 'chapel' was really the only visible and quite open sign of death inside the hospital area. Not least for me, an ordinary patient.

And I knew I had to see it. Sooner or later.

Many people may die every day at Ullevål hospital. I myself know people who died there. But the only trace of death I saw was this concrete ramp. Now I had seen it.

It calmed me in some way.

Chapter Four

So now I was to regard myself as cured. Several people had told me so; that it was important to 'decide' that you were cured when the treatment was over.

It would not be true to say I felt any special sense of being cured. I did not really feel ill, but an infinite emptiness descended on me. I also stopped going to the physiotherapist, as there was little more she could do for me now that I couldn't do for myself with a few daily exercises. So I now had to face everyday life.

I did not expect to find it so difficult. I began to see to what extent I had clung to that fixed routine, the daily trip to Ulleval and three times a week to the physiotherapist. All that had been my crutches. Now the crutches were gone and I had to walk all by myself!

The woman doctor had told me that most people go through depressions with this disease, and she had added that those who go back into some activity as soon as possible managed the best.

That sounded sensible. But I was in no condition to sit down at my desk and go on working on the book I had been writing when I was first told about the cancer in February. I was in no state to sit down at my desk and produce articles for newspapers, either. I was empty. I was exhausted.

I thought along these lines – if I had been employed somewhere, and had been able to go to work, where someone would give me work to do, then undoubtedly, I would be able to do it. But my job consists of giving myself work, finding subjects of interest about which to write. I had a dreadful sense of *no one* and *nothing* interesting me. A terrible, all-engrossing self-absorption had settled on my whole life.

What should I do? I asked myself.

'Take your time,' said my closest friend. And I did. For the first time in my life, I think, I took my time.

This tremendous self-absorption that follows on after an illness like breast cancer, which at heart is raw self-pity, is in the long run sterile. I had read about animals like cats and elephants for instance, that, when about to die, go and hide themselves in isolation, away from all the others. There is certainly something of the animal in us, which leads to this self-absorption which arises during illness. But although the animal in us, our instincts if you like, are important, they are not enough. Alone, you are narrow and sterile, and 'the others', from whom you retreat, are necessary to life. And 'the others' are those closest to you, from whom I had also retreated – friends, family, acquaintances – as well as 'the world' for that matter, in the sense that my profession centred on it so much.

In the long run, this instinctive solitude is self-pity, a lifeless desert. There comes a point when you feel that either you will sink down into it, or drift into an existence where you become a kind of object, officially alive, but really dead. Dead in your soul, because all contact is broken except what is relevant to your illness.

One day I felt I had reached some kind of dangerous borderline, where I could either slide in behind the invisible milestone, or else I would have to turn and gather my strength to make my way back to 'the others'.

'You must regard yourself as cured,' a doctor had said to me on the telephone, in what seemed to me was a young and vigorous voice. And that is certainly true.

A great deal, in ourselves as well as in this fatal thing called illness, is a question of will-power, the will to live, the ability to look things in the eye and live for the moment. It was not that certain that I had been so terribly ill, either. 'Cancer Mammae' can clearly be everything or nothing. A gamble really.

But I kept an intense watch on my own need for illusions, my ability to live a lie. Take the worst as an utterly real possibility, I kept repeating to myself. Why? Because I knew I would not be able to stand a shock of the kind I had received in February, 1983, when I was told I had cancer.

I would plumb my own terror. If the best were to be my destiny, and I 'wanted to be alive in twenty years' time', as another doctor had expressed it, then this life would be a unique gift to me. And if not, then I would in some way adapt myself to death, and the possibility would no longer be allowed to shock me.

But this is easier said than done. I have noticed that people with faith, whether Christians, Moslems or Jews – or Marxists and Leninists for that matter, who also have faith within a structure of history – that all 'believers' had a kind of ultimate triumph with which to face death, anyway in the abstract.

Maybe there is a paradise waiting for them, a fatherland and refuge – or they may believe they will bring an earthly utopia to the world in a storm-cloud of fire and blood and 'truth'.

But what can a poor thing who simply feels that such beliefs are fantasies do? I am probably a typical child of my day in that I take the advance of knowledge for what it is and cannot really get around it. That is also a form of belief, of course. If I am to be slightly more concrete, then I would say I actually 'believe' that mankind, and that also includes myself, is a product of 'chance and necessity', as the French biologist and Nobel prizewinner, Jacques Monod, once expressed it.

We are really a microscopic cog in a gigantic machine, which, for us anyway, is meaningless, in the sense that the ultimate meaning of the universe and life is not mankind. But at the same time, I know that we human beings have the ability to see ourselves from the outside, and to admit to this infinite loneliness in a universe that appears blind and ice-cold to us. I also know that inbuilt in ourselves, so to speak, in the genetic code of which each one of us is a result, we clearly have a persistent need for an explanation of life and a meaning in life.

In this respect, I presumably differ from the blue-

117

tits at my window to a greater extent than I differ from Christians, Moslems, Jews and Marxist-Leninists. Animals probably do not know of their loneliness, while we carry our loneliness within us in the form of an obsessive anguish, and out of our anguish, since time immemorial we have created more and more sophisticated explanations, myths, religious and social systems of 'sacred' kinds.

I think I can say that none of these creations of ours constitute the truth for me. I am a creature of the twentieth century and the worm has eaten so much of the old faith in me, that there is now nothing left but the peel. But I sense the primaeval wisdom about ourselves and our lives stored in all these religions and systems. So I am not 'anti-religion', provided religions are not used in the eternal game of power and oppression.

But I feel I am at bedrock, and that is where I meet mankind, my brother and sister, that creature who is also myself.

What do I see there? Apart from religions and systems, or to be more exact the *basis* of them, I see our ability and need to *express* ourselves. Just look at it, in the form of images, notes, words and physical movements! We use that all-embracing and generalized expression – art.

We are creative beings. That is bedrock for me.

It is a fairly solid standpoint, at least that is how I see it. I am convinced that this creative ability and the need to create in our species will produce new 'solutions' to the riddle of life, new forms of faith, if you like, which make it possible for us to survive our own pride and desire for power.

That is only what I believe, but I am not excluding the possibility that our species may commit suicide in its phrenetic and arrogant belief that it is chosen by God or History, the first-born, the wonderful crown-jewel in the magnificent crown of the universe.

I had no choice. I *had* to take my time. But I also felt I was at a crossroads. I had to get out of this sterile world of self-absorption. I had to wriggle my way out of the power my illness had over me. In some way, I had to get back to 'the others', those close to me and to the world outside.

This was where I instinctively tried to find what I call bedrock.

So much of what one seizes on at such moments is chance. Antonio Vivaldi, the composer, was one of those musicians I had had a slightly special feeling for ever since I had seen a television series in France a few years earlier, a series on and by the Venetian chamber orchestra, *I Solisti Veniti*, conducted by Claudio Scimone, who had specialized in Vivaldi's music and the instruments of Vivaldi's day.

The programme had been recorded in Venice, with all its canals and its strange border country between sea and city, and in it the ancient houses and flying gulls were interwoven with the playing of the musicians and Vivaldi's music.

The programme had impressed me, and so I bought a set of cassettes of Vivaldi's music recorded by that particular orchestra. I now took out those cassettes. Not 'The Four Seasons' primarily, Vivaldi's best known work, at least in Norway. His concertos for mandolin, that instrument so typical of Vivaldi's day and Venice, were my first choice, as well as his concerto for 'violin discordato', as it is called in Italian. Vivaldi had caught my interest because of his free and light rhythms, his eternal allegros, as you might say.

At this particular time, he gradually came to mean very much more to me. His allegros were no longer just lighthearted, triumphant cascades of notes creating an instant atmosphere. So much lay beneath the 'triumphant' notes, a richness that included everything inside you, that weeps right through the 'joie de vivre' and 'triumphs'. In all his elegant and bell-like mandolin notes and his sweeping, rushing strings, there is an undertone of the anguish we human beings always carry with us, with a zest for life, in fact, so much more profound than the dark notes that are always there to emphasize the light.

I could not hear these Vivaldi concertos without seeing the French television programme before me. They were the first really good music programmes I had ever seen on television. What I saw all the time, as the notes poured out into my apartment in Vika, was the gulls soaring above the canals of Venice – soaring gulls, looping in towards a burning sun on the lagoons of Venice, soaring gulls in among the ancient houses of Venice. Birds – birds and notes, sun and sea and ancient city streets.

I have a special feeling for gulls.

Not just those hooded-gulls that settle in the Palace Park in Oslo, for instance, nor the gulls swarming round garbage tips outside cities. It is the great black-backed gulls I feel specially for. I have spent every summer for the last eleven years, as well as at other times of the year, by the sea at Ryfylke, with those majestic great black-backed gulls as daily and close companions.

I smelt the sea and seaweed, almost felt myself to

be a gull soaring away on my mighty wings round some of the lonely isles and skerries, and letting myself sail on the wind in over the land. One of the few 'andantes' by Vivaldi, in one of his mandolin concertos, caught hold of my boundless self-pity and transformed it into – well, what did it transform it into?

This is what is so remarkable about art, about beauty, that what is most sterile within you is brought out into the light, and suddenly you feel the blood streaming through you in a kind of joy beyond grief. What is it that is so remarkable about art, this fantasy product which you have not even produced yourself, but which you receive in a way as if it had sprung from your own self?

The gulls became a signal for me, and one day something extraordinary happened to me.

I was walking through the Arts Society in Kjell Stub Street in Oslo, where they had an exhibition of ceramics by thirteen potters from eight countries, made by what was called the 'Kecskemet Group'. It did not attract me very much first time round. The ceramics were interesting experiments with materials of all kinds . . . but then – a white bird. A gull's head upraised and the faintest inklings of wings trying to spread.

I stood rooted to the spot. I identified myself with this porcelain sculpture in a way I found it hard to explain. There was a whole series of these birds, some in white porcelain with touches of black, others in brilliant colours. They were made by Kari Christensen, a potter of whom in my ignorance I had never heard.

Of course I don't know what this artist had herself 'meant' with these birds, but I know I was one

121

of them, struck down in some way, imprisoned in something that prevented me from flying, and what tenderness there was in this artist's portrayal of this free and imprisoned bird, this vulnerable creature. It was the same as in Vivaldi, the grief and self-pity in me, the anguish, too, were taken from me, and were there in this delicate porcelain shape before my eyes.

I did something I have very rarely allowed myself to do in my life, nor could I really afford it – I bought the bird on the spot. I was, of course, not allowed to take it home until after the end of the exhibition several weeks later, but I had a photograph in the catalogue of a similar bird. I knew the bird would not leave me. One day I would be able to carry it back to Vika and put it in my room.

Music, porcelain, notes, I felt them creeping in on me and sweeping a mist away from my inner landscape, just as the sun does on summer seaside mornings, when the warmth of its rays dissolves the mist standing like a wall outside your window.

When the mist had lifted, the desire to tackle words began to rise in me. I am no musician, nor sculptor, nor potter. I am a person of words.

I have been writing for as long as I can remember – all my life. I have always written. But words had been impossible for me over this period of time. Then one day I came across a sentence in Jacques Mondo's book *Chance and Necessity*, on page 111 – (it is nonsense that the selection process is decisive to the development of man) –

' . . . an impartial observer, a Martian, for instance, would undoubtedly have to admit that the development of the specific human achievement, symbolic language – a unique event in the biosphere – opened the way for another development, which created a totally new power, namely that of culture, thought and perception.'

I know that. If we human creatures are a jewel of some species, then it is our 'symbolic language', the words we use, that have to answer for such a belief. We are less silent than animals. With words, we rise out of ourselves and can perceive ourselves and the world around us, and with them we can reach 'the others'.

One day, I sat down at my typewriter. It is a lovely machine, a brand-new electronic typewriter. But I hadn't touched it since last February. I sat down cautiously in the middle of my study, pulled out the machine on its low trolley, plugged it in and put in a clean piece of paper.

What would I write? I would write IT. I suddenly knew quite clearly. I would just go ahead with no real plan. Not tell a story. Not bring a message. I would just write my way through all the weeks I had been through and which now lay like a thick mist over my mind.

I knew suddenly, with a kind of ecstasy, that for me there was fundamentally only one thing of any value, apart from being alive, and that was to be able to sit down in my room and write.

I started. I started just as this short book starts: 'It never occurred to me that it could happen to me'. I looked at that line and thought – right. That's the truth. It had never occurred to you that you were a brittle, vulnerable creature, who in addition has never

ever been promised anything special.

No. I pushed all that away. I would stick to the facts. I would simply take it day by day . . .

That is what I have done. I have now written my way through those weeks. I am not saying I have written down everything. I have been selective. There are many things that are not easy to talk about, and I have kept off my private life. As the French writer Colette says: 'Ce n'est pas que je me cache, mais je n'aime pas me montrer'. (It's not that I hide away, but that I don't like to show myself.)

With a bundle of typewritten pages, I went off to Ryfylke, my gulls and my sea, and sat finishing it off as it ends here.

Now that I have completed it, I feel that the way to 'the others' has opened up again. The mist has lifted. Under any circumstances, I have crafted a piece of work. That's what writing is, a craft.

This craft work in itself is a good enough explanation for why it is practised. The craft of writing is to bring us nearer to each other, and to lead us on to the way to perception.

84 CHARING CROSS ROAD

Helene Hanff

'Unmitigated delight from cover to cover'
DAILY TELEGRAPH

First published in the UK in 1971, 84 CHARING CROSS
ROAD has now become something of a classic, more
recently increasing its wide circle of fans when it was
seen in a London stage adaptation. It is the very simple
story of the love affair between Miss Helene Hanff of New
York and Messrs Marks and Co, sellers of rare and
secondhand books, at 84 Charing Cross Road, London.

'Immensely appealing . . . witty, caustic'
LISTENER

'20 years of faithful and uproarious correspondence with
a bookshop in Charing Cross Road'
EVENING STANDARD

'A lovely read, a must for all who worship books'
BOOKS AND BOOKMEN

Futura Publications
Non-Fiction
0 8600 7438 2

PLAIN TALES FROM THE RAJ

Edited by Charles Allen

The bestselling collection of reminiscences of British India that is based upon the famous Radio 4 series.

'One of the most enjoyable books I have read . . . by turns informative, funny and deeply touching. It is an authentic record of the survivors of British India . . . a book which takes on where Kipling takes off'
ANTONIA FRASER

'That extraordinary world of crows and dust sunsets, of dinner parties that started with anchovy toast (always) and ended seven courses later with little glass bowls full of water and hibiscus flowers to wash the fingers in; of cane chairs on club verandahs, and damp sugar full of ants; of shining Indian rivers and beautiful women . . . Pure nostalgia and irresistible'
SCOTSMAN

'Britons ruled for almost three centuries creating a society the like of which will never be repeated. The flavour of the era is captured in PLAIN TALES FROM THE RAJ'
DAILY MIRROR

Futura Publications
Non-Fiction/Autobiography
0 8600 7455 2

THE CORNCRAKE AND THE LYSANDER

Finlay J Macdonald

'Wit, irony and laughter . . . triumphant'
GLASGOW HERALD

THE 30s WERE GROWING TO A CLOSE. FOR THE ISLAND
OF HARRIS, THE WORST YEARS OF THE DEPRESSION
WERE OVER.

As Finlay Macdonald set out from his tiny village for high
school in Tarbert, Hitler's growing military strength had
begun to menace the people of Europe. But to Finlay the
coming fray was just one more exciting prospect along
with living in Big Grandfather's house, making new friends
and meeting the beautiful girls of his adolescent dreams.

And as the rasping croak of the elusive corncrake was
drowned out by the moan of the protective Lysander plane,
Finlay's adventures brought him much laughter — but
there were also tears as the pride of the island's young
men sailed off to battle, many never to return.

Don't miss Finlay Macdonald's CROWDIE AND CREAM
and CROTAL AND WHITE, also available from Futura.

Futura Publications
Non Fiction/Autobiography
0 7088 2776 4

All Futura Books are available at your bookshop or
newsagent, or can be ordered from the following address:
Futura Books, Cash Sales Department,
P.O. Box 11, Falmouth, Cornwall.

Please send cheque or postal order (no currency), and
allow 55p for postage and packing for the first book plus
22p for the second book and 14p for each additional book
ordered up to a maximum charge of £1.75 in U.K.

Customers in Eire and B.F.P.O. please allow 55p for the
first book, 22p for the second book plus 14p per copy for
the next 7 books, thereafter 8p per book.

Overseas customers please allow £1 for postage and
packing for the first book and 25p per copy for each
additional book.